Practical Phlebology

Deep Vein Thrombosis

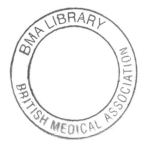

Practical Phlebology

Series Editors: Lowell S. Kabnick, Neil S. Sadick

PUBLISHED

Practical Phlebology: Starting and Managing a Phlebology Practice
Marlin Schul; Saundra Spruiell; Clint Hayes
2010 • ISBN 9781853159404

Practical Phlebology: Venous Ultrasound
Joseph Zygmunt; Olivier Pichot; Tracie Dauplaise
2013 • ISBN 9781853159404

Practical Phlebology: Deep Vein Thrombosis
Anthony J. Comerota
2014 • ISBN 9781444146480

Practical Phlebology

Deep Vein Thrombosis

Anthony J. Comerota

Series Editors:

Lowell S. Kabnick MD FACS
Associate Professor of Surgery, New York University,
Langone Medical Center, New York; and
Director, NYU Vein Center, NY, USA

Neil S. Sadick MD FAAD FAACS FACPH
Clinical Professor of Dermatology,
Weill Cornell Medical College,
Cornell University, New York, NY, USA

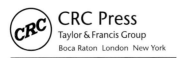

CRC Press
Taylor & Francis Group
Boca Raton London New York

CRC Press is an imprint of the
Taylor & Francis Group, an **informa** business

CRC Press
Taylor & Francis Group
6000 Broken Sound Parkway NW, Suite 300
Boca Raton, FL 33487-2742

© 2014 by Taylor & Francis Group, LLC
CRC Press is an imprint of Taylor & Francis Group, an Informa business

No claim to original U.S. Government works

Printed on acid-free paper
Version Date: 20130919

International Standard Book Number-13: 978-1-4441-4609-7 (Hardback)

This book contains information obtained from authentic and highly regarded sources. While all reasonable efforts have been made to publish reliable data and information, neither the author[s] nor the publisher can accept any legal responsibility or liability for any errors or omissions that may be made. The publishers wish to make clear that any views or opinions expressed in this book by individual editors, authors or contributors are personal to them and do not necessarily reflect the views/opinions of the publishers. The information or guidance contained in this book is intended for use by medical, scientific or health-care professionals and is provided strictly as a supplement to the medical or other professional's own judgement, their knowledge of the patient's medical history, relevant manufacturer's instructions and the appropriate best practice guidelines. Because of the rapid advances in medical science, any information or advice on dosages, procedures or diagnoses should be independently verified. The reader is strongly urged to consult the drug companies' printed instructions, and their websites, before administering any of the drugs recommended in this book. This book does not indicate whether a particular treatment is appropriate or suitable for a particular individual. Ultimately it is the sole responsibility of the medical professional to make his or her own professional judgements, so as to advise and treat patients appropriately. The authors and publishers have also attempted to trace the copyright holders of all material reproduced in this publication and apologize to copyright holders if permission to publish in this form has not been obtained. If any copyright material has not been acknowledged please write and let us know so we may rectify in any future reprint.

Library of Congress Cataloging-in-Publication Data

Comerota, Anthony J. , author.
    Practical phlebology. Deep vein thrombosis / Anthony J. Comerota.
    p. ; cm. -- (Practical phlebology)
    Deep vein thrombosis
    Includes bibliographical references and index.
    ISBN 978-1-4441-4609-7 (hardback : alk. paper)
    I. Title. II. Title: Deep vein thrombosis. III. Series: Practical phlebology.
    [DNLM: 1. Venous Thrombosis. WG 610]

RC697
616.1'45--dc23   2013036986

Visit the Taylor & Francis Web site at
http://www.taylorandfrancis.com

and the CRC Press Web site at
http://www.crcpress.com

Dedication

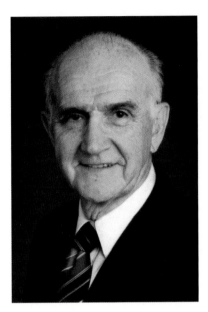

"Tony ... ALWAYS DO WHAT'S RIGHT!"

John J. Cranley
1918–2003

Contents

Series Preface

It is with great pleasure and enthusiasm that I introduce the latest volume of the Practical Phlebology manual series, *Practical Phlebology: Deep Vein Thrombosis*. When the series was first conceptualized with the Royal Society of Medicine, we outlined a number of potential volumes to be authored by leading international phlebological experts. These volumes were to be published as and when each volume was completed. Since the release of the first-in-series manual in 2010, *Starting and Managing a Phlebology Practice*, and our 2013 volume, *Venous Ultrasound*, published by our new publishing company CRC Press, we have taken the opportunity to review the planned volume titles and scope of the series. We take pleasure in announcing our next volume will be *Minimally Invasive Surgery and Sclerotherapy*.

We would like to thank CRC Press, Claire Bonnett, and her expert staff who support and facilitate the Practical Phlebology series.

Lowell S. Kabnick, MD
Neil S. Sadick, MD

Foreword

The precise number of people affected by DVT in the United States is unknown; however, most estimates of this serious problem reach 600,000 patients per year. Each year DVT involves 1 to 2 people per 1,000, and in those over 80 years of age these numbers can reach as high as 1 in 100 people. Alarmingly, in 25% of DVT patients the first symptom is sudden death, 10 to 30% of people will die within one month of diagnosis, and of the survivors approximately 50% will have long-term complications in the affected limb.

Once again the Practical Phlebology series would be remiss not to include a dedicated manual to DVT. We are extremely fortunate to have as the author of our DVT volume, Anthony Comerota, MD. He is "Mr. DVT." As many of you are aware and for those who are not, Dr. Comerota has contributed to many of the adopted medical and surgical guidelines for managing DVT. Hopefully, you will benefit from his hard work, as I have. With the author's wisdom, experience and expertise, this manual is invaluable for the venous practitioner.

Lowell Kabnick, MD
NYU Langone Medical Center
Vascular and Endovascular Surgery Division
and
Director, NYU Vein Center
New York, New York

Preface

This book on acute deep vein thrombosis (DVT) is written for clinicians so that they may have a better understanding of the disease process and its etiology and a current review of optimal patient care. It is also written for the academician. The material included is based upon pertinent peer-reviewed literature and good quality clinical trials that serve to illuminate proper clinical decision making. Needless to say, this subject is fertile ground for ongoing basic and clinical research.

This book begins with the epidemiology and natural history of acute DVT, which itself may be a misnomer, as most of the observations of the "natural history" of acute DVT have been in patients receiving anticoagulation. The book ends with a strong suggestion to the reader that "not all DVTs are the same."

The etiology of DVT follows. I took the opportunity to review some of the insightful work of Dr. Gwendolyn Stewart, who I had the distinct privilege of working with early in my career. As part of the Sol Sherry Thrombosis Research Center at Temple University Health Sciences Center, we investigated venodilation and endothelial damage as etiologic factors of acute DVT in animals and appropriate clinical investigation in humans. The observations were compelling, although this element of pathophysiology is seldom recognized.

If we in the medical profession had completely effective DVT prophylaxis, and if it were used uniformly, this text would be substantially abbreviated. Current recommendations are specifically addressed in Chapter 3 on DVT prophylaxis.

Diagnosis of acute DVT is quite reliable today, although definitive diagnostic techniques are not always available 24 hours a day. Therefore, other, less definitive diagnostic and treatment algorithms need to be adopted.

The remainder of the book addresses treatment in its many forms. While anticoagulation is the mainstay, strategies of thrombus removal have been shown to be superior to anticoagulation alone for the management of iliofemoral DVT. We await the results of the ATTRACT trial to confirm those of CaVenT (for iliofemoral DVT) and to report whether catheter-based interventions and thrombolysis are more effective than anticoagulation alone in reducing postthrombotic syndrome in patients with femoropopliteal DVT. Inferior vena cava filters and heparin-induced thrombocytopenia are also covered in separate chapters. I hope the readers enjoy the "white clot" as it appears upon removal from blood vessels.

Although the final chapter, "Common femoral endovenectomy and endoluminal recanalization for chronic postthrombotic iliofemoral venous obstruction," does not formally fall under the heading of acute DVT, I thought I must include it. It illustrates to readers that the long-term morbidity of extensive thrombus that remains within the vein is due to obliteration (obstruction) of venous return from the leg by the thrombus evolving to a fibrous occlusion, which is overwhelmingly collagen. While it is possible to reduce the severe postthrombotic syndrome in these patients by this relatively new but infrequently performed procedure, it is far easier and more effective to treat the acute thrombotic event with an appropriate strategy of thrombus removal.

In closing, I acknowledge the extreme patience and support of my wife, Elsa. The dedicated editorial assistance of Marilyn Gravett has lightened the load of putting this text together. The graphic expertise of Kurt Mansor is deeply appreciated. Claire Bonnett and her expert staff at CRC Press have smoothly advanced the entire process in a professional and friendly manner.

Finally, I dedicate this book to my former mentor, the late Dr. John J. Cranley, of Cincinnati, Ohio, who had a lifelong interest in venous disease. Dr. Cranley was a mentor and inspiration to many. He was a leader by example, a man dedicated to God, his family, and friends, and a person who never took advantage of his position for self-gain. His guiding principle was "Always do what's right!" Although he mainly used this saying referring to patient care, all those who knew him understood that it was a simple motto by which he lived. I have long been and will continue to be guided by his example.

About the Author

Anthony J. Comerota, MD, FACS, FACC, director of the Jobst Vascular Institute at Toledo Hospital, Toledo, Ohio, and adjunct professor of surgery at the University of Michigan, received his medical degree from Temple University School of Medicine in Philadelphia, Pennsylvania, and completed his general surgery residency at Temple University Hospital and his vascular surgery fellowship at Good Samaritan Hospital, Cincinnati, Ohio.

Dr. Comerota returned to the Temple University Health Sciences Center as a faculty member, where he became chief of vascular surgery, professor of surgery, program director in general and vascular surgery, president of the medical staff, and president of the Medical Alumni Association. In 2002, Dr. Comerota accepted his present position.

Dr. Comerota has been a major contributor to the development of some of the newest forms of treatment for vascular disease and has been the principal investigator of seven major national trials and a co-investigator of numerous others. His research interests span a broad range of arterial and venous disorders, including the management of acute DVT, therapeutic angiogenesis, noninvasive diagnosis of vascular disease, development of new devices, new drug development, and the effects of platelet-inhibiting drugs. He has received over $5 million in research funding, including support from the National Institutes of Health (NIH), the American Heart Association, and the American Diabetes Association.

Dr. Comerota has had a special interest in venous disease. He has investigated the etiology of acute DVT, DVT prophylaxis, mechanical and hematologic effects of compression, and strategies of thrombus removal to prevent postthrombotic syndrome. Dr. Comerota has served as the president of the American Venous Forum, the venous section editor of the Vascular Self Assessment Program of the Society for Vascular Surgery, and has been a member of the guideline writing committees for the treatment of venous thromboembolism of the American College of Chest Physicians and the International Union of Angiology.

Dr. Comerota is a member of 20 professional societies and has served as president of four major societies. He is an associate editor for *Vascular*, sits on the editorial board of *Vascular and Endovascular Surgery* and *Annals of Vascular Surgery*, and is a reviewer for 17 other journals, including the *New England Journal of Medicine*. Dr. Comerota has written or edited 7 textbooks and has authored or coauthored more than 300 publications.

Dr. Comerota is a member of the Alpha Omega Alpha Honorary Society and honorary fellow of the Royal Australasian College of Surgeons, the Japanese Society of Phlebology, and the European Venous Forum. He has received the Alumni Merit Award from Millikin University and been named to Who's Who in America and Best Doctors in America.

Natural history of acute DVT

Overview

The goal of treating deep vein thrombosis (DVT) is to prevent pulmonary embolism (PE) and death from PE, reduce the risk of recurrent DVT, and avoid postthrombotic morbidity. To manage DVT optimally, an understanding of its natural history is important. It is helpful to conceptualize venous thrombosis as an imbalance of the patient's coagulation system with the fibrinolytic system at the time of the acute event and over the long term. Anticoagulation is designed to shift this imbalance toward the patient's endogenous fibrinolytic system to reduce endovenous coagulation. If the patient's fibrinolytic system is capable of resolving the majority of the acute clot, postthrombotic morbidity will be reduced and potentially avoided. However, if the effectiveness of the fibrinolytic system is minimal or if thrombus extension or rethrombosis occurs, the likelihood of additional venous thromboembolic complications and postthrombotic morbidity is high.

The clinical presentation of the patient and the natural history of thrombus evolution depend upon the anatomic distribution, the extent of the blood clot, and the degree of occlusion of the involved veins. Patients who have isolated calf vein thrombosis generally have fewer postthrombotic symptoms and higher rates of successful thrombus resolution with anticoagulation than those with femoropopliteal DVT.[1,2] Likewise, patients with femoropopliteal DVT do not have the same severity of postthrombotic morbidity as patients with iliofemoral DVT.[2] Considering that the common femoral vein, external iliac vein, and common iliac veins are the single venous outflow channel for the entire lower extremity, one would expect that occlusion of that outflow channel would lead to the most severe postthrombotic morbidity. This is the case, as demonstrated by natural history studies focused on patients with iliofemoral DVT and a prospective study of postthrombotic morbidity.[3-6]

In addition to the extent and location of the thrombus, the etiology of the thrombus plays an important role also. Patients who have a transient high risk resulting in thrombosis, such as those undergoing an operative procedure, have different outcomes and long-term prognosis compared to those who develop idiopathic DVT.[7-13]

DVT and mortality

Perhaps not surprising, mortality after acute DVT is increased compared to age-matched controls. The in-hospital case fatality rate for acute DVT is approximately 5%. Subsequent 1-, 3-, and 5-year mortality rates of 22%, 30%, and 39%, respectively, have been reported.[14-16] Cancer is the most common cause of early death in patients with acute DVT,[15,17] especially in patients over 44 years of age. The 1-month mortality rate among cancer patients with DVT is as high as 25%,[18] and the 1-year mortality rate is reported as high as 63%,[15] compared to 12.6% in patients without cancer. The duration of increased risk for mortality in patients with DVT and cancer persists for at least 3 years, if not more, after diagnosis, whereas the mortality risk following secondary DVT (transient risk) returns to that of the general population after 6 months.[15]

Venous thrombotic complications are linked to arterial thrombotic events, specifically cardiovascular death. Since acute thrombosis is the common denominator of both DVT and myocardial infarction (and death from myocardial infarction), it is not surprising that the presence of residual venous thrombus at the time anticoagulants are discontinued following treatment for acute DVT may be a marker for a cardiovascular event.[19,20] There appears to be a definite association between idiopathic venous thromboembolic events and clinical cardiovascular disease. Patients with idiopathic venous thromboembolism (VTE) were found to have more atherosclerotic risk factors than control subjects with VTE,[21] and the 10-year risk of a symptomatic cardiovascular event among patients with idiopathic DVT was 25.4% compared with 12.9% in those with a secondary venous thromboembolic event.[22]

Thrombus resolution

Ideally, thrombus resolution would occur in all patients treated for DVT, thereby restoring vein patency and preserving valve function. Some recanalization of venous thrombi occurs in the majority of patients. Killewich et al.[23] showed that 86% of patients developed some recanalization within 3 months of initial thrombosis. Van Ramshorst et al.[24] likewise showed that 87% of patients with femoropopliteal DVT developed recanalization of occluded segments within 6 weeks. Tibial thrombi generally clear more rapidly, which may reflect the larger surface area of endothelium to thrombus volume, thereby improving efficiency of fibrinolysis in small veins.

The amount of recanalization that occurs is inversely correlated with the degree of activated coagulation and fibrinolytic inhibition.[25,26] When observed clinically, older patients, veins with smaller thrombi, and nonocclusive thrombi have more effective recanalization and thrombus resolution than occluded veins and patients with multisegment venous thrombosis. Therefore, the initial volume of thrombus predicts the degree of recanalization. What is suggested but has not been confirmed is whether the thrombus burden is related to the level of activated coagulation factors and plasminogen activator inhibition (PAI).

DVT, valve function, and recurrence

In his classic work, Sevitt[27,28] demonstrated that thrombosis often originated in the area of venous valves. While his work is frequently quoted, most fail to recognize that while the thrombus may surround the valve, often it is not attached to the valve cusp, but rather is attached to the vein wall above or below the valve. This suggests that there are functional differences of the endothelium covering the valve leaflet compared to the endothelium covering the vein wall.

This specific issue has been studied by Brooks et al.,[29] who studied the venous endothelium on the vein wall adjacent to a vein valve cusp and the endothelium covering the valve in human saphenous veins. They demonstrated that endothelial protein C receptor activity and thrombomodulin (antithrombotic proteins) were present in significantly higher concentrations on the valve than the adjacent vein wall, and that von Willebrand factor (a procoagulant) was present in higher concentrations on vein wall endothelium than vein valve endothelium. These observations fit well with the ultrasound correlations of Killewich et al.,[23] Markel et al.,[30] and Meissner et al.,[31] and help to explain their observations that rapid thrombus resolution preserved vein valve function. In these studies, rapid thrombus resolution was defined as occurring within 2 to 3 months of diagnosis. Resolution that occurred beyond that time often resulted in valvular incompetence. This suggests that the valve leaflet is entrapped by the thrombus, and once fibrous attachment of the thrombus to a vein wall occurs and the leaflet is encompassed by the thrombus, the leaflet will no longer function, as it will be retracted with the fibrotic evolution (retraction) of the thrombus. On the other hand, if thrombus resolution occurs early, valve leaflets can return to normal function since thrombus was not attached to the valve cusp initially.

Pathophysiology of postthrombotic morbidity

Venous valvular dysfunction and venous obstruction are the two main components leading to ambulatory venous hypertension. Ambulatory venous hypertension is the underlying pathophysiology causing chronic venous disease and the postthrombotic syndrome.[32,33] While venous valvular function is easy to identify and can be precisely quantified, venous obstruction often remains undiagnosed. Current invasive and noninvasive studies fail to adequately identify venous obstruction, and venous obstruction cannot be quantified. Therefore, there is widespread underappreciation of the importance of venous obstruction as a contribution to postthrombotic morbidity (Figure 1.1). However, when obstruction is recognized, patients generally have significant postthrombotic symptoms, and when obstruction and valve incompetence are found in the same patients, postthrombotic morbidity is severe.[32,34]

A well-recognized risk factor for postthrombotic morbidity is ipsilateral recurrent thrombosis. Venous thrombosis has been shown to recur in up to 24% of patients at 5 years and 30% of patients at 8 years following initial diagnosis.[20,35,36] It is recognized that patients with idiopathic DVT or thrombophilia have a 2.5- to 3-fold increased risk of recurrence compared to patients with transient risk factors.

The adequacy of anticoagulation during the course of treatment for acute DVT is associated with recurrent events. Subtherapeutic anticoagulation early in the treatment of acute DVT is associated with a 15-fold increased risk

of recurrence. During the long-term course of therapy, the risk of new thrombotic events increases 1.4-fold for each 20% reduction in time of therapeutic anticoagulation.[37,38]

Persistent luminal obstruction and thrombus activity are important elements factoring into the risk of recurrent thrombosis. Following termination of anticoagulation, failure of complete recanalization manifested by persistent luminal obstruction on duplex ultrasound was associated with a significantly higher risk of recurrence compared to patients with a normal duplex examination.[35,36,39] Furthermore, ongoing thrombus activity demonstrated by elevated D-dimer levels 1 month after anticoagulation is discontinued has been shown to be associated with a 310% increased risk of recurrent thrombosis.[40,41]

Not all DVTs are the same

Unfortunately, to many physicians all DVT is the same, and all are treated with anticoagulation alone. There are important subsets of patients that define their natural history, recurrence rates, and postthrombotic morbidity. As reviewed earlier in this chapter, idiopathic DVT has a worse prognosis than DVT associated with a transient high-risk factor. Importantly, the level of venous

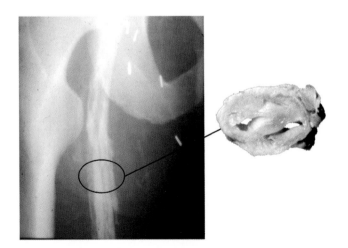

Figure 1.1 Chronic postthrombotic venous disease in a patient who had iliofemoral DVT treated with anticoagulation 10 years earlier. An ascending phlebogram showed recanalization of the iliofemoral venous system; radiologic assessment was that there was "no obstruction" and a 3-second maximal venous outflow test was "normal." After a classic Linton procedure was performed, a cross section of the femoral vein documented relatively extensive luminal obstruction.

system involvement and whether the clot is occlusive versus nonocclusive will be important predictors of recurrence and postthrombotic morbidity.[1,3,5,14]

Calf vein thrombosis

Patients with *isolated calf vein thrombosis* are generally viewed as having the least severe thrombus burden and the best prognosis. Although PE can occur, the emboli are generally small and often asymptomatic. Thrombus resolution occurs in many, if not most, of these patients when treated with anticoagulation.[1,26] A randomized trial has shown that thrombus extension and recurrence occurs in up to 19% of patients who are not treated compared to no major thromboembolic complications observed in patients anticoagulated for 3 months.[2] Current guidelines recommend anticoagulation for 3 months in patients with isolated calf vein thrombosis.[42]

Femoral vein thrombosis

Patients with *isolated femoral vein thrombosis*, especially thrombus limited to the segment of vein in the mid or upper thigh, generally do well with anticoagulation alone. The profunda femoris vein offers good collateral venous drainage from the popliteal to the common femoral, and the patients often have functional valves above and below the vein segment involved with thrombus. Whether recanalization of the thrombus occurs or not is not particularly important as long as the popliteal and common femoral veins remain free of clot.

Popliteal vein thrombosis

Patients who have *popliteal vein thrombosis*, which occludes the popliteal "trifurcation," often have severe acute symptoms and are at risk of significant postthrombotic morbidity. When the axial venous drainage of the calf is occluded, patients have severe distal venous hypertension. Although this is an infrequent and unique subset of patients, they have a high likelihood of severe postthrombotic morbidity. In this subset of patients who

are active, I will consider thrombolysis to restore venous patency and reduce their postthrombotic morbidity.

Iliofemoral DVT

Iliofemoral DVT is a clinically relevant subset of patients. Since the iliofemoral venous segment represents the single outflow tract from the entire lower-extremity venous system, it is intuitive that when obstructed, severe postthrombotic morbidity will follow.

Table 1.1 shows the morbidity of iliofemoral DVT patients who are treated with anticoagulation alone, summarized from two natural history studies.[5,6] Although these observations were made at 5 years, patients generally are severely symptomatic from the time of their acute event onward.

Qvarfordt and Eklof[43] measured compartment pressures in patients with acute iliofemoral DVT before and after venous thrombectomy. They demonstrated exceptionally high compartment pressures while the venous outflow tract was obstructed, with return to normal after venous thrombectomy. Persistently high venous pressures lead to the postthrombotic syndrome, venous claudication, and the consequences of chronic venous disease.

In a prospective analysis of patients with acute DVT treated with anticoagulation, Kahn et al.[3] demonstrated a significantly higher risk of severe postthrombotic syndrome in patients with iliofemoral DVT compared with those with infrainguinal venous thrombosis.

It is well established that ipsilateral recurrent DVT increases the risk of postthrombotic syndrome as much as sixfold. Douketis et al.[44] demonstrated that patients with iliofemoral DVT had a

Table 1.1 Iliofemoral DVT treated with anticoagulation

Observations
• 95% develop venous insufficiency
• 15% develop venous ulceration
• Venous claudication results in 40%
• Limited ambulation results in 15%
• Marked hemodynamic impairment occurs in most
• Markedly reduced quality of life occurs in most

Sources: Akesson H, et al., *Eur J Vasc Surg* 1990; 4:43–48; Delis KT, et al., *Ann Surg* 2004; 239:118–126.

Table 1.2 Natural history of acute DVT: key observations

1. Idiopathic DVT has greater morbidity and recurrence rates than secondary (transient risk factor) DVT.
2. The extent of thrombosis and number of venous segments involved determine postthrombotic morbidity.
3. Persistent venous obstruction and thrombus activity are associated with increased recurrence.
4. Iliofemoral DVT is associated with severe postthrombotic morbidity.
5. Iliofemoral DVT is associated with significantly higher recurrence rates.

significantly higher risk of recurrence compared to those with infrainguinal thrombosis. This is likely to be due to the greater amount of venous obstruction and higher level of persistent thrombus activity following iliofemoral DVT.

Considering the body of evidence to date regarding the natural history of acute DVT treated with anticoagulation, a number of key observations have been made (Table 1.2).

REFERENCES

1. Killewich LA, Macko RF, Cox K, et al. Regression of proximal deep venous thrombosis is associated with fibrinolytic enhancement. *J Vasc Surg* 1997; 26:861–868.
2. Lagerstedt CI, Olsson CG, Fagher BO, Oqvist BW, Albrechtsson U. Need for long-term anticoagulant treatment in symptomatic calf-vein thrombosis. *Lancet* 1985; 2: 515–518.
3. Kahn SR, Shrier I, Julian JA, et al. Determinants and time course of the postthrombotic syndrome after acute deep venous thrombosis. *Ann Intern Med* 2008; 149:698–707.
4. O'Donnell TF, Browse NL, Burnand KG, Thomas ML. The socioeconomic effects of an iliofemoral venous thrombosis. *J Surg Res* 1977; 22:483–488.
5. Akesson H, Brudin L, Dahlstrom JA, et al. Venous function assessed during a 5 year period after acute ilio-femoral venous thrombosis treated with anticoagulation. *Eur J Vasc Surg* 1990; 4:43–48.
6. Delis KT, Bountouroglou D, Mansfield AO. Venous claudication in iliofemoral thrombosis: long-term effects on venous hemodynamics, clinical status, and quality of life. *Ann Surg* 2004; 239:118–126.
7. Prandoni P, Lensing AW, Cogo A, et al. The long-term clinical course of acute deep venous thrombosis. *Ann Intern Med* 1996; 125:1–7.
8. Prandoni P, Villalta S, Bagatella P, et al. The clinical course of deep-vein thrombosis. Prospective long-term follow-up of 528 symptomatic patients. *Haematologica* 1997; 82:423–428.
9. Hansson PO, Sorbo J, Eriksson H. Recurrent venous thromboembolism after deep vein thrombosis: incidence and risk factors. *Arch Intern Med* 2000; 160:769–774.
10. Heit JA, Silverstein MD, Mohr DN, et al. Risk factors for deep vein thrombosis and pulmonary embolism: a population-based case-control study. *Arch Intern Med* 2000; 160:809–815.
11. Prandoni P, Noventa F, Ghirarduzzi A, et al. The risk of recurrent venous thromboembolism after discontinuing anticoagulation in patients with acute proximal deep vein thrombosis or pulmonary embolism. A prospective cohort study in 1,626 patients. *Haematologica* 2007; 92:199–205.
12. Deitcher SR, Kessler CM, Merli G, et al. Secondary prevention of venous thromboembolic events in patients with active cancer: enoxaparin alone versus initial enoxaparin followed by warfarin for a 180-day period. *Clin Appl Thromb Hemost* 2006; 12:389–396.
13. Eichinger S, Weltermann A, Minar E, et al. Symptomatic pulmonary embolism and the risk of recurrent venous thromboembolism. *Arch Intern Med* 2004; 164:92–96.
14. Beyth RJ, Cohen AM, Landefeld CS. Long-term outcomes of deep-vein thrombosis. *Arch Intern Med* 1995; 155:1031–1037.

15. Naess IA, Christiansen SC, Romundstad P, et al. Incidence and mortality of venous thrombosis: a population-based study. *J Thromb Haemost* 2007; 5:692–699.

16. Anderson FA Jr., Wheeler HB, Goldberg RJ, et al. A population-based perspective of the hospital incidence and case-fatality rates of deep vein thrombosis and pulmonary embolism. The Worcester DVT Study. *Arch Intern Med* 1991; 151:933–938.

17. Cushman M, Tsai AW, White RH, et al. Deep vein thrombosis and pulmonary embolism in two cohorts: the longitudinal investigation of thromboembolism etiology. *Am J Med* 2004; 117:19–25.

18. White RH. The epidemiology of venous thromboembolism. *Circulation* 2003; 107: 14–18.

19. Savory L, Harper P, Ockelford P. Posttreatment ultrasound-detected residual venous thrombosis: a risk factor for recurrent venous thromboembolism and mortality. *Curr Opin Pulm Med* 2007; 13:403–408.

20. Young L, Ockelford P, Milne D, et al. Post-treatment residual thrombus increases the risk of recurrent deep vein thrombosis and mortality. *J Thromb Haemost* 2006; 4:1919–1924.

21. Hong C, Zhu F, Du D, et al. Coronary artery calcification and risk factors for atherosclerosis in patients with venous thromboembolism. *Atherosclerosis* 2005; 183:169–174.

22. Prandoni P, Ghirarduzzi A, Prins MH, et al. Venous thromboembolism and the risk of subsequent symptomatic atherosclerosis. *J Thromb Haemost* 2006; 4:1891–1896.

23. Killewich LA, Bedford GR, Beach KW, Strandness DE Jr. Spontaneous lysis of deep venous thrombi: rate and outcome. *J Vasc Surg* 1989; 9:89–97.

24. Van Ramshorst B, Van Bemmelen PS, Hoeneveld H, Faber JA, Eikelboom BC. Thrombus regression in deep venous thrombosis. Quantification of spontaneous thrombolysis with duplex scanning. *Circulation* 1992; 86:414–419.

25. Meissner MH, Zierler BK, Bergelin RO, Chandler WL, Strandness DE Jr. Coagulation, fibrinolysis, and recanalization after acute deep venous thrombosis. *J Vasc Surg* 2002; 35:278–285.

26. Arcelus JI, Caprini JA, Hoffman KN, et al. Laboratory assays and duplex scanning outcomes after symptomatic deep vein thrombosis: preliminary results. *J Vasc Surg* 1996; 23:616–621.

27. Sevitt S. The structure and growth of valve-pocket thrombi in femoral veins. *J Clin Pathol* 1974; 27:517–528.

28. Sevitt S. The mechanisms of canalisation in deep vein thrombosis. *J Pathol* 1973; 110:153–165.

29. Brooks EG, Trotman W, Wadsworth MP, et al. Valves of the deep venous system: an overlooked risk factor. *Blood* 2009; 114:1276–1279.

30. Markel A, Meissner M, Manzo RA, Bergelin RO, Strandness DE Jr. Deep venous thrombosis: rate of spontaneous lysis and thrombus extension. *Int Angiol* 2003; 22:376–382.

31. Meissner MH, Manzo RA, Bergelin RO, Markel A, Strandness DE Jr. Deep venous insufficiency: the relationship between lysis and subsequent reflux. *J Vasc Surg* 1993; 18:596–605.

32. Shull KC, Nicolaides AN, Fernandes e Fernandes J, et al. Significance of popliteal reflux in relation to ambulatory venous pressure and ulceration. *Arch Surg* 1979; 114:1304–1306.

33. Nicolaides AN, Schull K, Fernandes E. Ambulatory venous pressure: new information. In Nicolaides AN, Yao JS (eds.), *Investigation of vascular disorders*. New York: Churchill Livingstone, 1981: 488–494.

34. Johnson BF, Manzo RA, Bergelin RO, Strandness DE Jr. Relationship between changes in the deep venous system and the development of the postthrombotic syndrome after an acute episode of lower limb deep vein thrombosis: a one- to six-year follow-up. *J Vasc Surg* 1995; 21:307–312.

35. Prandoni P, Lensing AW, Prins MH, et al. Residual venous thrombosis as a predictive factor of recurrent venous thromboembolism. *Ann Intern Med* 2002; 137:955–960.

36. Lindmarker P, Schulman S. The risk of ipsilateral versus contralateral recurrent deep vein thrombosis in the leg. The DURAC Trial Study Group. *J Intern Med* 2000; 247:601–606.

37. Caps MT, Meissner MH, Tullis MJ, et al. Venous thrombus stability during acute phase of therapy. *Vasc Med* 1999; 4:9–14.

38. Hull RD, Raskob GE, Hirsh J, et al. Continuous intravenous heparin compared with intermittent subcutaneous heparin in the initial treatment of proximal-vein thrombosis. *N Engl J Med* 1986; 315:1109–1114.

39. Prandoni P, Prins MH, Lensing AW, et al. Residual thrombosis on ultrasonography to guide the duration of anticoagulation in patients with deep venous thrombosis: a randomized trial. *Ann Intern Med* 2009; 150:577–585.

40. Eichinger S, Minar E, Bialonczyk C, et al. D-dimer levels and risk of recurrent venous thromboembolism. *JAMA* 2003; 290:1071–1074.

41. Palareti G, Cosmi B, Legnani C, et al. D-dimer testing to determine the duration of anticoagulation therapy. *N Engl J Med* 2006; 355:1780–1789.

42. Kearon C, Kahn SR, Agnelli G, et al. Antithrombotic therapy for venous thromboembolic disease: ACCP evidence-based clinical practice guidelines (8th ed). *Chest* 2008; 133:454S–545S.

43. Qvarfordt P, Eklof B, Ohlin P. Intramuscular pressure in the lower leg in deep vein thrombosis and phlegmasia cerulae dolens. *Ann Surg* 1983; 197:450–453.

44. Douketis JD, Crowther MA, Foster GA, Ginsberg JS. Does the location of thrombosis determine the risk of disease recurrence in patients with proximal deep vein thrombosis? *Am J Med* 2001; 110:515–519.

2

Etiology

Overview

Deep venous thrombosis (DVT) and pulmonary embolism (PE) are considered part of the same pathophysiologic state termed *venous thromboembolism*. This remains a common problem if not an increasing problem in the United States.[1] Improved methods of diagnostic testing as well as the aging of our population are important reasons for its increasing prevalence.

It is estimated that approximately 1 million people are diagnosed with DVT each year. Approximately 300,000 die of a venous thromboembolic complication, which exceeds that of acute myocardial infarction or acute stroke.[1]

Factors that may contribute to the high incidence of venous thromboembolic complications are: (1) an aging population, putting more patients at risk; (2) operative procedures being performed on higher-risk patients; and (3) greater awareness of venous thromboembolic complications with increased use of improved diagnostic procedures.

Although DVT and PE are considered part of the same clinical pathologic process, the remainder of this monograph will focus on DVT of the lower extremities.

Etiology

The factors responsible for venous thrombosis in the absence of direct vein wall injury have been of interest for more than a century. In 1856, Rudolf Ludvig Karl Virchow,[2] the father of cellular pathology, proposed his classic triad elucidating the etiology of venous thrombosis (Figure 2.1). He indicated that changes in blood elements (hypercoagulability), reduced blood flow velocity (stasis), and vein wall injury (endothelial damage) combined to produce an environment promoting thrombus formation (Figure 2.2). These concepts remain true today; however, our contemporary view is fashioned by our increased knowledge and understanding of blood coagulation, molecular and cellular biology, the body's response to injury, and genetics.

Stasis

It is widely accepted that stasis can be a factor leading to DVT. Radiographic demonstrations (ascending phlebograms) as well as radionucleotide studies have demonstrated that venous stasis occurs in surgical patients.[3,4] This author believes that stasis is a "permissive factor" for DVT rather than a causative factor. In the presence of vein wall injury or a procoagulant state, stasis permits thrombosis to occur more frequently than in patients without stasis. However, there are no studies showing that in otherwise normal conditions, stasis alone will result in thrombosis.

A classic autopsy study by Gibbs[5] demonstrated that soleal sinuses are the principal site of origin of venous thrombosis. Since the soleal sinuses have been the areas of most profound stasis, a natural conclusion was that stasis was a causative factor for DVT. Although evidence indicates that stasis occurs, it is logical that reduced flow velocity prolongs contact time of activated platelets and clotting factors with the vein wall, thereby permitting thrombus formation. These observations fit with the findings of subsequent research by Stewart et al.[6]

Hypercoagulability

Although *procoagulant state* appears to be a better term than *hypercoagulability*, hypercoagulability or thrombophilia is used as a result of convention. The effect of procoagulant states and the existence of stasis were investigated in surgical patients by Stead[7] and Hirsh et al.[8] They demonstrated that an increased risk of thrombosis was associated with increased plasma procoagulant activity in surgical patients, including increases in platelet counts and adhesiveness, and changes in the coagulation cascade, such as an increase in clotting factors

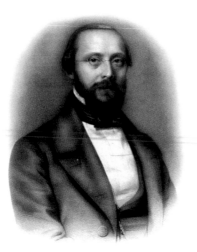

Figure 2.1 Photograph of Professor Rudolph Virchow, father of cellular pathology.

and a decrease in endogenous fibrinolytic activity. Deficiencies in antithrombin III, protein C, protein S, and plasminogen, as well as the presence of a circulating lupus anticoagulant, pointed to either a primary or secondary procoagulant state.

Advances in cellular and molecular biology will help us understand the link between procoagulant states, stasis, and thrombosis. This is predominantly through studies investigating vascular inflammation and thrombosis. Stewart et al.[6] initially suggested that there was a relationship between inflammation and thrombosis. She demonstrated with scanning electron microscopy the activation and adhesion of leukocytes and platelets to the vein wall, suggesting that these may be initiating factors of vein wall damage. Research has demonstrated that inflammatory mediators upregulate procoagulant factors and downregulate natural anticoagulants and endogenous fibrinolysis.

While it is beyond the scope of this text to review in detail the advances in cellular and molecular biology as they contribute to thrombosis, it is important to put into context the initiating steps of venous thrombosis as clearly defined by the elegant research performed within the last 20 years. Understanding these steps will translate into improved prophylaxis and treatment.

To understand the molecular and cellular contributions, it is important to recognize the link between selectin biology, white blood cells, platelets, and the presence and effects of microparticles. White blood cell adhesion to vascular endothelium is controlled by the binding of vascular selectins to leukocytes.[9]

Selectins are a family of glycoproteins that are expressed on the surface of white blood cells, platelets, and endothelial cells. They are important in

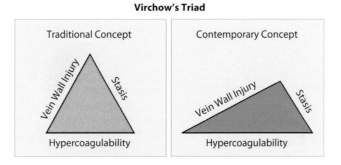

Figure 2.2 Virchow's triad: traditional and contemporary concepts.

leukocyte and platelet rolling over the endothelium and their adhesion to areas of vascular injury and the subsequent inflammatory response that develops. Three selectins have been described: L-selectin, E-selectin, and P-selectin. The majority of the work in this area has focused on P-selectin.

P-selectin is important in the rolling and initial adhesion of platelets and white blood cells to areas of endothelial injury.[10] Furthermore, animal models have demonstrated that P-selectin activity regulates fibrin deposition and thrombus size.[11,12] Microparticles are small phospholipid vesicles that are released from platelets, leukocytes, and endothelial cells.[13-15] Although microparticles are normal constituents of blood, their protein expression profile depends upon their cell of origin, and their protein and phospholipid content determines their biologic activity. Microparticles rich in certain phospholipids are potent substrates for coagulation.

Animal studies have demonstrated that when microparticles bind to activated platelets, tissue factor is released and thrombosis is initiated.[16] White blood cells (monocytes) are capable of concentrating tissue factor and P-selectin ligand. When monocytes bind to areas of tissue injury, microparticles are released that deliver tissue factor-promoting inflammation, further activating platelets, resulting in the generation of fibrin.[17]

Animal models of vein wall injury have demonstrated that microparticles play a crucial role in stasis-induced thrombosis with small vascular injury.[18] Furthermore, microparticles are not only prothrombotic but also inhibit endogenous fibrinolysis by releasing platelet activator inhibitor-1 (PAI-1).[19]

Vein wall injury

The procoagulant state and stasis factors of Virchow's triad have been put into perspective by the contemporary cellular and molecular research summarized previously. However, the role of vein wall injury in the initiation of thrombosis has received relatively little attention, despite evidence that vein wall injury occurs distant from the site of trauma. There is little argument that direct injury to a vein wall leads to thrombus formation. However, when observing the problem of postoperative DVT, it is clear that veins distant from the site of an operation (calf veins) are the most common site of postoperative DVT, yet most are not directly damaged during the operative procedure.

In order to study that endothelial damage occurred distant from a site of an operation, animal models were developed. These models investigated large abdominal operations as well as total hip replacement in canine experiments.[20,21] Schaub and coworkers found that leukocytes adhered to and invaded the wall of jugular and femoral veins along their entire length following abdominal surgery.[20] They theorized that these endothelial lesions distant from the operative site were induced by products of tissue injury that were released at the wound and gained entry into the circulation (Figure 2.3). It was subsequently demonstrated that mild venous endothelial damage occurred after abdominal operations and that more severe endothelial damage was found after total hip replacement.[21] Scanning electron microscopic examinations (Figure 2.4a–e) showed endothelial tears located around the junctions of small side

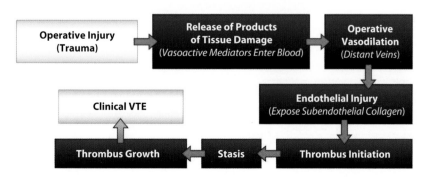

Figure 2.3 Concept of operative trauma causing distant venous endothelial injury.

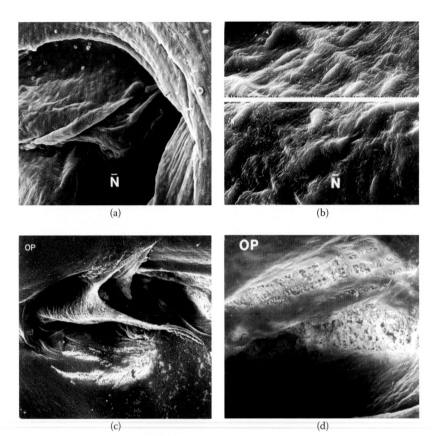

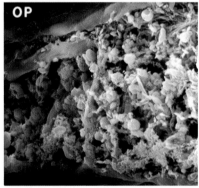

Figure 2.4 Scanning electron micrograph of the intimal surface of the jugular vein of a dog that was anesthetized but did not receive an operation. The ostium of a side branch is centered, with a valve (V) visualized. Both low-power (a) and high-power (b) magnification demonstrate an intact endothelial monolayer without evidence of damage. The electron micrographs of the jugular vein of a dog that underwent total hip replacement (OP) and had significant operative venodilation. Note that under low-power magnification (c), an endothelial tear (t) is located in the area of a valve cusp (v). With progressively higher magnification, it appears that the endothelial damage occurred as a stretching (tearing) mechanism. The damage extends through the endothelium and basement membrane, exposing highly thrombogenic subendothelial collagen (d). With higher-power magnification, one observes the attachment of red blood cells, white blood cells, platelets, and fibrin strands to the area of vein wall damage, indicating the initiation of thrombosis (e).

branches to the jugular and femoral veins.[22] These tears extended through the endothelium and the basement membrane, exposing subendothelial collagen, which is known to be highly thrombogenic. These lesions were then rapidly infiltrated with leukocytes and platelets, resulting in fibrin deposition and the initiation of thrombus. The constant location of the endothelial damage was interesting in that it was on the vein wall adjacent to a valve cusp, which was in the area of a side branch. The vein wall immediately adjacent to a side branch is attenuated with marked reduction in smooth muscle and connective tissue,[23] making it particularly susceptible to vein wall injury.

It was postulated that the products of tissue injury produced at the site of the operation caused operative venodilation that might result in the initial intimal damage. Stewart and colleagues[24] then demonstrated that dilation of the jugular vein beyond a certain point correlated with an increased frequency of venous endothelial lesions observed in their canine model. Interestingly, the femoral veins appeared more susceptible to operative venodilation than did the jugular veins in the frequency of endothelial lesions observed.[25]

There is substantial clinical evidence supporting the theory that operative venodilation is a cause of postoperative DVT in humans. If one examines the human studies of DVT prophylaxis, observations made by Kakkar and associates,[26] the Multicenter Trial Committee,[27] and Beisaw and colleagues[28] have demonstrated that the addition of a venotonic agent, dihydroergotamine, to low-dose heparin

significantly reduced postoperative DVT. Therefore, there appeared to be a link between the clinical observation in humans and the experimental observation in laboratory animals. This led to clinical studies that evaluated the impact of operative venous dilation on postoperative DVT in patients undergoing total hip and total knee replacement and to determining whether preventing operative venodilation prevented postoperative DVT.

In the first study, patients undergoing total hip replacement were randomized to receive dihydroergotamine plus heparin or placebo in a blinded fashion, and all patients had the diameter of their cephalic vein (contralateral to the operated hip) continuously monitored during the operation (Figure 2.5).[29] Ascending phlebography was performed in all patients postoperatively to assess for DVT. Results showed a significant difference in venodilation between patients who had postoperative DVT and those who did not. Interestingly, patients with excessive operative venodilation were older than patients with minimal or no dilation. This points to the link between age, venous pathophysiology, and subsequent thrombosis. Patients who developed postoperative DVT had significantly greater dilation and were significantly older than patients in whom DVT did not occur. There was a clear threshold at which it appeared the venodilation produced a degree of injury that uniformly resulted in thrombosis. All patients whose veins dilated more than 20% of their baseline diameter developed postoperative DVT, irrespective of age. On the other hand, only 17% of

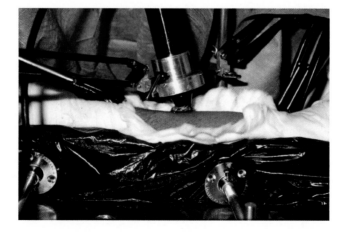

Figure 2.5 Operative photograph of contralateral cephalic vein being monitored with B-mode ultrasound during total hip replacement.

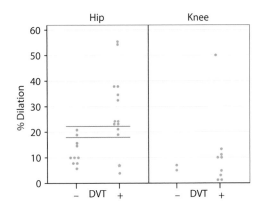

Figure 2.6 Graph of results correlating operative venodilation with postoperative phlebograms. Note that the majority of patients developing DVT following hip replacement sustained significant operative venodilation, whereas no patient (except one outlier) undergoing total knee replacement had operative venodilation in excess of 15%.

patients whose veins dilated less than 20% developed postoperative DVT ($p < .002$). The patients who received a venotonic agent had a significant reduction of operative venodilation and a significantly reduced incidence of postoperative DVT. As mentioned before, age was a risk factor for operative venodilation and postoperative DVT.

In the second study of patients undergoing total knee replacement,[30] operative venodilation was not observed (except for one outlier) (Figure 2.6). Although there was a high incidence of ipsilateral postoperative DVT, no patient developed contralateral DVT, whereas a substantial number of patients undergoing total hip replacement develop contralateral postoperative DVT. Because total knee replacements are performed with the use of a thigh tourniquet (creating regional circulatory arrest), products of tissue injury do not gain entry into the systemic circulation during the operation, and operative venodilation therefore should not (and does not) occur. On the other hand, high concentrations of these metabolic by-products in the wound and surrounding tissues lead to local venous injury, resulting in ipsilateral postoperative DVT.

These observations of operative venodilation occurring in patients undergoing total hip replacement but not occurring in patients having total knee replacement have clinical relevance. Total hip replacement patients have an appreciable incidence of DVT contralateral to the hip operated,

whereas DVT in total knee replacement patients is uniformly confined to the operated leg. These clinical correlations linked to the observations of operative venodilation in total hip and total knee patients unify the etiologic theories of venous thrombosis. The observations that operative venodilation occurs in humans have been confirmed by Coleridge-Smith and coworkers.[31]

More than 150 years after Virchow's initial description of the factors leading to venous thrombosis, the observations remain valid. Our understanding has been expanded by the cellular and molecular biologic research and clinical observations reported by contemporary and prior investigators.

REFERENCES

1. Heit JA, Cohen AT, Anderson FA Jr., on behalf of the VTE Impact Assessment Group. Estimated annual number of incident and recurrent, non-fatal and fatal venous thromboembolism (VTE) events in the US. *ASH Ann Meeting Abstr* 2005; 106:910.
2. Virchow R. Neuer Fall von todlicher Emboli er Lungenarterie. *Arch Pathol Anat* 1856; 10:225.
3. Clark C, Cotton LT. Blood-flow in deep veins of leg. Recording technique and evaluation of methods to increase flow during operation. *Br J Surg* 1968; 55:211–214.
4. Nicolaides AN, Kakkar VV, Renney JT. Soleal sinuses and stasis. *Br J Surg* 1971; 58:307.
5. Gibbs NM. Venous thrombosis of the lower limbs with particular reference to bed-rest. *Br J Surg* 1957; 45:209–236.
6. Stewart GJ, Ritchie WG, Lynch PR. Venous endothelial damage produced by massive sticking and emigration of leukocytes. *Am J Pathol* 1974; 74:507–532.
7. Stead RB. The hypercoagulable state. In Goldhaber SZ (ed.), *Pulmonary embolism and deep venous thrombosis*. Philadelphia: W.B. Saunders, 1985: 161.
8. Hirsh J, Barlow GH, Swann HC, Salzman EW. Diagnosis of pre-thrombotic state in surgical patients. *Contemp Surg* 1980; 16:65.
9. Tedder TF, Steeber DA, Chen A, Engel P. The selectins: vascular adhesion molecules. *FASEB J* 1995; 9:866–873.

10. Subramaniam M, Frenette PS, Saffaripour S, et al. Defects in hemostasis in P-selectin-deficient mice. *Blood* 1996; 87:1238–1242.

11. Wakefield TW, Strieter RM, Downing LJ, et al. P-selectin and TNF inhibition reduce venous thrombosis inflammation. *J Surg Res* 1996; 64:26–31.

12. Palabrica T, Lobb R, Furie BC, et al. Leukocyte accumulation promoting fibrin deposition is mediated *in vivo* by P-selectin on adherent platelets. *Nature* 1992; 359:848–851.

13. Gilbert GE, Sims PJ, Wiedmer T, et al. Platelet-derived microparticles express high affinity receptors for factor VIII. *J Biol Chem* 1991; 266:17261–17268.

14. Mesri M, Altieri DC. Endothelial cell activation by leukocyte microparticles. *J Immunol* 1998; 161:4382–4387.

15. Sabatier F, Roux V, Anfosso F, et al. Interaction of endothelial microparticles with monocytic cells *in vitro* induces tissue factor-dependent procoagulant activity. *Blood* 2002; 99:3962–3970.

16. Osterud B. The role of platelets in decrypting monocyte tissue factor. *Semin Hematol* 2001; 38:2–5.

17. Falati S, Liu Q, Gross P, et al. Accumulation of tissue factor into developing thrombi *in vivo* is dependent upon microparticle P-selectin glycoprotein ligand 1 and platelet P-selectin. *J Exp Med* 2003; 197:1585–1598.

18. Polgar J, Matuskova J, Wagner DD. The P-selectin, tissue factor, coagulation triad. *J Thromb Haemost* 2005; 3:1590–1596.

19. Booth NA, Simpson AJ, Croll A, Bennett B, MacGregor IR. Plasminogen activator inhibitor (PAI-1) in plasma and platelets. *Br J Haematol* 1988; 70:327–333.

20. Schaub RG, Lynch PR, Stewart GJ. The response of canine veins to three types of abdominal surgery: a scanning and transmission electron microscopic study. *Surgery* 1978; 83:411–424.

21. Stewart GJ, Alburger PD Jr., Stone EA, Soszka TW. Total hip replacement induces injury to remote veins in a canine model. *J Bone Joint Surg Am* 1983; 65:97–102.

22. Stewart GJ, Schaub RG, Niewiarowski S. Products of tissue injury. Their induction of venous endothelial damage and blood cell adhesion in the dog. *Arch Pathol Lab Med* 1980; 104:409–413.

23. Stone EA, Stewart GJ. Architecture and structure of canine veins with special reference to confluences. *Anat Rec* 1988; 222:154–163.

24. Stewart GJ. Personal communication. 1990.

25. Comerota AJ, Stewart GJ. Operative venous dilation and its relation to postoperative deep venous thrombosis. In Goldhaber SZ (ed.), *Prevention of venous thromboembolism*. New York: Marcel Dekker, 1993: 25–50.

26. Kakkar VV, Stamatakis JD, Bentley PG, et al. Prophylaxis for postoperative deep-vein thrombosis. Synergistic effect of heparin and dihydroergotamine. *JAMA* 1979; 241:39–42.

27. Dihydroergotamine–heparin prophylaxis of postoperative deep vein thrombosis. A multicenter trial. The Multicenter Trial Committee. *JAMA* 1984; 251:2960–2966.

28. Beisaw NE, Comerota AJ, Groth HE, et al. Dihydroergotamine/heparin in the prevention of deep-vein thrombosis after total hip replacement. A controlled, prospective, randomized multicenter trial. *J Bone Joint Surg Am* 1988; 70:2–10.

29. Comerota AJ, Stewart GJ, Alburger PD, Smalley K, White JV. Operative venodilation: a previously unsuspected factor in the cause of postoperative deep vein thrombosis. *Surgery* 1989; 106:301–308.

30. Stewart GJ, Lachman JW, Alburger PD, et al. Intraoperative venous dilation and subsequent development of deep vein thrombosis in patients undergoing total hip or knee replacement. *Ultrasound Med Biol* 1990; 16:133–140.

31. Coleridge-Smith PD, Hasty JH, Scurr JH. Venous stasis and vein lumen changes during surgery. *Br J Surg* 1990; 77:1055–1059.

3

DVT prophylaxis

Overview

Hospital-acquired venous thromboembolism (VTE) remains a major problem in the developed countries. In the United States it is estimated that over 1 million have a venous thromboembolic event annually.[1] Approximately 300,000 people die as a result of pulmonary embolism (PE), which exceeds deaths due to acute myocardial infarction (MI) or acute stroke. Most fatalities from PE occur early. Comparable estimates have been published evaluating data from the United Kingdom, France, Spain, Germany, Italy, and Sweden, which are countries with similar disease distribution and treatment patterns.[2] Since many patients present with nonspecific features, the diagnosis of PE is often missed. Another interesting fact is that less than 20% of patients who die from PE have the diagnosis of deep vein thrombosis (DVT) at the time of their fatal event. Therefore, one could conclude that 80% or more of fatal PEs occur as a result of *asymptomatic DVT*.

The spectrum of DVT (and VTE) is broad, and the complications of DVT are serious (Figure 3.1). Patients may develop symptomatic DVT generating a clinical suspicion that leads to diagnostic investigation. Once the diagnosis is made, appropriate treatment can be instituted. However, primary prophylaxis that avoids the biologic onset of venous thrombosis is the preferred management of high-risk patients. Prophylaxis has been shown to reduce mortality of PE and all-cause mortality.[3] Screening of high-risk patients with imaging techniques to identify asymptomatic DVT in preference to administering prophylaxis is generally not cost-effective. If symptomatic DVT occurs and is diagnosed, proper treatment can favorably affect outcome toward recovery, thereby avoiding disability and death.

Despite effective means of DVT prophylaxis being available for surgical and medically ill patients, PE remains the most common preventable cause of death in hospitalized patients. The risk of a venous thromboembolic event occurring after surgery in patients not receiving prophylaxis is summarized in Table 3.1. While the rates recorded in Table 3.1 are from studies reported 12 to 20 or more years ago, and operative techniques have improved along with patient ambulation, resulting in potentially lower inherent rates of postoperative DVT, fatal PE continues to be a major but preventable postoperative complication. Although fatal PE is recognized after surgical procedures and 10% of all hospital deaths are due to PE, VTE in hospitalized patients is not only a surgical problem.[4] Fifty to seventy percent of symptomatic venous thromboembolic events and 70% to 80% of fatal PEs occur in medical patients.[5] In a prospective study of medical ICU patients, DVT was detected by venous ultrasound in 33%.[6]

Risk stratification

Numerous risk factors have been identified over the years. As a result of a literature review, it is apparent that some risk factors are more potent than others. Therefore, in an effort to more accurately stratify risk, the concept of *risk factor equivalents* was applied to evaluate patients hospitalized at

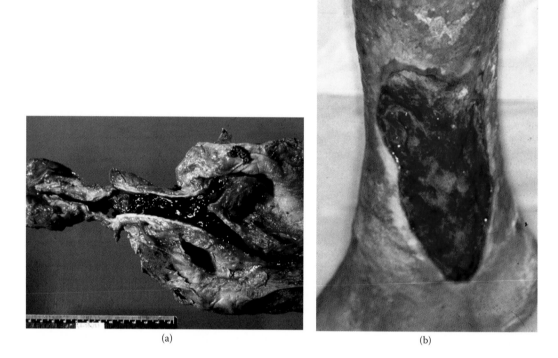

(a)   (b)

Figure 3.1 Complications of acute DVT include (a) pulmonary embolism (in this example, fatal) and (b) post-thrombotic syndrome (in this example, showing a patient with a venous ulcer).

Table 3.1 Risk of VTE without prophylaxis after surgery

Surgical procedure	Incidence of DVT
Knee surgery	75%
Hip fracture surgery	60%
Elective hip surgery	50%–55%
Retropubic prostatectomy	40%
General abdominal surgery	30%–35%
Gynecological surgery	25%–30%
Neurosurgery	20%–30%
Transurethral resection of prostate	10%
Inguinal hernia repair	10%

the Toledo Hospital and hospitals in the ProMedica Health System. Using this method of risk assessment, individual patient risk is evaluated, and each patient can have appropriate prophylaxis prescribed. These risk factors have been integrated into a VTE risk assessment tool for patients being hospitalized (Table 3.2). The proper method of prophylaxis depends upon the number of risk factors identified for each patient.

An important consideration for appropriate prophylaxis is the patients whose VTE risk increases during hospitalization, and therefore their prophylaxis changes. To identify these patients one must plan ongoing, repeated risk assessment. On busy nursing care units, this may be delayed or overlooked. If risk assessment is the responsibility of the physician, both initial and repeat assessments are less likely to occur.

Risk assessment and prophylaxis guidelines that are being implemented for nonorthopedic surgical and nonsurgical patients at this author's institution essentially divide patients into two groups, *low risk*, who require no additional prophylaxis other than early ambulation, and *high risk*, who will receive mechanical as well as pharmacologic prophylaxis. This approach offers appropriate prophylaxis to all high-risk patients and all moderate-risk patients whose risk profile increases.

Table 3.2 VTE risk assessment tool

Low risk (0–1) 1 risk factor equivalent	Moderate risk (2–4) 2 risk factor equivalents	High risk (≥5) 3 risk factor equivalents
Age 40–59	Age ≥ 60	History of DVT/PE
Bed confinement > 48 hours (history of or anticipated)	Trauma (reason for hospitalization)	Acute spinal cord injury (within past 6 weeks)
Varicose veins (observed or diagnosed)		Acute stroke
Any leg edema/ulcer/stasis	Joint replacement (admit Dx)	
Obesity (BMI ≥ 30)	Hip fracture (admit Dx)	
MI (current/past 2 weeks)	Malignancy (active)	
CHF (admit Dx)	Pelvic surgery (gynecological, colorectal, GU)	
Inflammatory bowel disease (admit Dx)	Pelvic/long-bone fracture (admit Dx)	
Crystalloids (>5 L/24 hours)	Hypercoagulable state (thrombophilia)	
Confining travel > 4 hours (within past 2 weeks)	Family history of DVT (siblings, parents, children)	
Pregnancy/postpartum (1 month)		
Severe COPD (admit Dx)		
Severe infection/sepsis		
Estrogen use (ERT and contraception)		
Operation > 2 hours duration (this hospitalization)		
Count boxes checked above	Count boxes checked above	Count boxes checked above
Multiply ×1	Multiply ×2	Multiply ×3
1st column total =	2nd column total =	3rd column total =
Risk score = sum of all three columns		

Note: BMI, body mass index; CHF, congestive heart failure; COPD, chronic obstructive pulmonary disease; DVT, deep vein thrombosis; Dx, diagnosis; ERT, estrogen replacement therapy; GU, genitourinary; MI, myocardial infarction; PE, pulmonary embolism; VTE, venous thromboembolism.

Moderate-risk patients may be overtreated according to the American College of Chest Physicians (ACCP) 2012 guidelines; however, we believe they will receive benefit and VTE events will be reduced in all patients. Our observation is that the most common error is underprophylaxis, which this approach is designed to avoid.

Interestingly, a recent hospitalization or a recent stay in a nursing home has been identified as a potent, independent risk factor for a venous thromboembolic event.[7] Although the majority of the patients diagnosed with DVT are outpatients, when investigated further, a large percentage were found to have had a recent hospitalization. It was found that many who developed DVT received inadequate or no DVT prophylaxis while in the hospital. It is intuitive that the mechanism for DVT in these patients was a medical or surgical illness requiring hospitalization, with inadequate inpatient prophylaxis leading to development of asymptomatic DVT while in the hospital. Postdischarge, the thrombus extends and enlarges to occlude the vein or embolize, subsequently becoming symptomatic and generating a diagnostic study resulting in the diagnosis of DVT or PE after discharge.

Prophylaxis guidelines

The ACCP has published practice guidelines for DVT prophylaxis for hospitalized patients.[8-10] The key guidelines are summarized in Tables 3.3–3.5. Every hospital should develop a strategy for VTE prophylaxis, and upon admission, all patients receive a risk assessment for VTE so that appropriate prophylaxis is prescribed.

Once the level of risk is established, the suggested options for proper prophylaxis are listed in Tables 3.4 and 3.5, and the attending physician can easily choose the appropriate option according to guidelines. The most recent ACCP guidelines have stratified recommendations for prophylaxis according to patient groups such as nonorthopedic surgical patients, orthopedic patients, and those with thrombophilia and pregnancy. These guidelines indicate that low-molecular-weight heparin (LMWH) be used in preference to other pharmacologic agents in orthopedic patients. Emerging data indicate that the combination of mechanical prophylaxis with effective pharmacologic prophylaxis offers the lowest risk of venous thromboembolic complications and is recommended by the ACCP in the highest-risk patients.[8,10]

The 2012 practice guidelines recommend that patients at high risk of bleeding receive graduated compression stockings or intermittent pneumatic compression (IPC) at a grade 2CA level.[8-10] One criticism of these guidelines is that compression stockings and IPC are considered as one method

Table 3.3 Key ACCP guidelines for VTE prevention in nonsurgical patients

Recommendation	Grade
For patients at low risk, no pharmacologic or mechanical prophylaxis is recommended	1B
For patients at increased risk of thrombosis, pharmacologic prophylaxis with LMWH, low-dose unfractionated heparin (LDUH) (b.i.d.), and LDUH (t.i.d.) for fondaparinux	1B
For patients at increased risk of thrombosis and high risk for major bleeding, mechanical prophylaxis is suggested	2C
In outpatients with cancer who have no additional risk factors for VTE, routine prophylaxis with LMWH, LDUH, or vitamin K antagonist (VKA) is not recommended	2B/2B/1B

Source: Data from Kahn SR, et al., *Chest* 2012; 141:e195S–e226S.

Table 3.4 Key ACCP guidelines for VTE prevention in nonorthopedic surgical patients

Recommendation	Grade
For very low-risk patients, no pharmacologic or mechanical prophylaxis is suggested other than early ambulation	2C
For low-risk patients, mechanical prophylaxis is suggested	2C
For moderate-risk patients not at high bleeding risk, LMWH, LDUH, or mechanical prophylaxis is recommended	2B 2B 2C
For high-risk patients not at high risk for bleeding, pharmacologic prophylaxis with LMWH or LDUH is recommended with the addition of mechanical compression	1B 2C
For patients at high risk for VTE undergoing abdominal or pelvic operations for cancer, extended-duration (4 weeks) pharmacologic prophylaxis with LMWH is recommended	1B
For patients at high risk of bleeding, mechanical prophylaxis is recommended	2C
For patients in all risk groups, it is suggested that an inferior vena cava (IVC) filter not be used for primary prophylaxis	2C

Source: Data from Gould MK, et al., *Chest* 2012; 141:e227S–e277S.

Table 3.5 Key ACCP guidelines for VTE prevention in orthopedic surgical patients

Recommendation	Grade
For patients undergoing major orthopedic surgery, LMWH, fondaparinux, dabigatran, apixaban, rivaroxaban, LDUH, adjusted-dose VKA, and aspirin (ASA) are recommended for a minimum of 10–14 days	1B
IPC is recommended in orthopedic surgery patients for a minimum of 10–14 days	1C
LMWH is suggested in preference to other agents	2C 2B
In patients receiving pharmacologic prophylaxis, IPC is suggested during the hospital stay	2C
Extended prophylaxis to 35 days is suggested	2B
In patients at increased risk of bleeding, IPC is recommended	2C
Use of an IVC filter is not suggested for primary prevention in patients with contraindication to pharmacologic or mechanical prophylaxis, or both	2C
Ultrasound screening before hospital discharge is not recommended	1B
For patients undergoing knee arthroplasty who do not have a history of VTE, no thromboprophylaxis is suggested	2B

Source: Data from Gould MK, et al., *Chest* 2012; 141:e227S–e277S.

BOX 3.1   MECHANISMS OF VTE PROPHYLAXIS OF INTERMITTENT PNEUMATIC COMPRESSION

1. Increases venous blood flow velocity (reduces stasis)[12]
2. Increases arterial perfusion[15]
3. Increases endogenous fibrinolytic activity (reduces hypercoagulability)[13]
4. Increases tissue factor pathway inhibitor and decreases factor VIIa[14]

---

and similarly effective, when in fact they are fundamentally different. The strength of this recommendation and hopefully separation of stockings and IPC as mechanical forms of prophylaxis will change, as the recent CLOTS trial has shown no benefit from graduated compression stockings in patients suffering acute stroke.[11] Since many experts believe that IPC offers more advantages than graduated compression stockings, and the underlying mechanisms leading to their effect are different (Box 3.1),[12–15] future guidelines will likely separate these two forms of mechanical prophylaxis.

Another important consideration is the patient who continues to be at high risk following hospital discharge. Current guidelines suggest that these patients continue to receive thromboprophylaxis with LMWH for up to 28 days following discharge. Hull et al.[16] recently reported the results of the EXCLAIM study. Over 4000 medical patients who were at high risk at discharge were randomized to receive either LMWH or placebo for 28 days. There was a 44% risk reduction in all venous thromboembolic events ($p = .001$), a 73% risk reduction in symptomatic VTE events ($p = .004$), and a 34% reduction in asymptomatic VTE ($p = .032$) in patients receiving extended prophylaxis. When calculating the number needed to treat and harm of treatment, 46 patients required treatment in order to avoid 1 VTE event, whereas treatment of 224 patients would result in 1 major bleeding event.

Bergqvist et al.[17] performed a similar study of high-risk cancer surgery patients called the ENOXACAN II trial. Patients were randomized at hospital discharge to receive either placebo or enoxaparin at 40 mg/day for 28 days. Prophylaxis resulted in a 60% relative risk reduction of VTE events ($p < .02$). These studies draw attention to the importance of postdischarge prophylaxis in high-risk medical and surgical patients, although aside from the high-risk surgical cancer patient and orthopedic patient, no postdischarge prophylaxis is recommended by ACCP 2012.

The type of prophylaxis has been studied in numerous trials. Comparisons of LMWH with unfractionated heparin (UFH) have been performed. In a recent meta-analysis of 36 trials evaluating LMWH versus UFH, Wein et al.[18] demonstrated a 32% risk reduction in VTE events in patients receiving LMWH versus UFH. The properties of LMWH appear particularly well suited for DVT prophylaxis and treatment and are reviewed in Chapter 5. As pharmacologic technology advanced, smaller compounds (such as the LMWHs) have been produced, ultimately resulting in the production of the pentasaccharide (fondaparinux). This parenteral compound indirectly inhibits (through binding with antithrombin) factor Xa. Randomized trials of fondaparinux with enoxaparin in patients undergoing orthopedic surgery for either total hip replacement, total knee replacement, or fractured hip have demonstrated that patients receiving fondaparinux had a 55% odds reduction of a VTE event and a 57.4% risk reduction of developing proximal DVT (Figure 3.2).[19-22] An important safety consideration when using fondaparinux for prophylaxis is to delay the first injection for 8 or more hours after completion of the operation. This significantly reduces postoperative bleeding without reducing efficacy. If fondaparinux is delayed ≥8 hours after the operation, it offers significant advantage over LMWH in orthopedic patients.

Combined mechanical and pharmacologic prophylaxis with fondaparinux was studied in the APOLLO trial of high-risk patients undergoing general surgery. Over 800 patients were randomized to receive IPC alone or IPC plus fondaparinux. Patients receiving combination therapy had a 1.7% incidence of postoperative VTE compared to 5.3% in patients receiving IPC alone. While there was a higher risk of major bleeding in the combination group (1.6% vs. 0.2%, $p = .006$), no bleeding episode was fatal or involved a critical organ. Similar to trials in orthopedic surgery, the timing of postoperative fondaparinux administration correlated with bleeding complications. Few bleeding complications occurred in patients receiving fondaparinux 8 or more hours postoperatively, whereas the majority of the bleeding complications occurred in patients receiving fondaparinux <6 hours after the operation was completed. The favorable results in APOLLO indicate the additive, if not synergistic, beneficial effect of combining mechanical with pharmacological prophylaxis.

Despite the volume of information available on the effectiveness of VTE prophylaxis, national studies have shown that 40% of surgical patients and 60% of medical patients fail to receive appropriate prophylaxis in the United States.[23] International trials likewise have demonstrated similar results whereby 50% or fewer of hospitalized patients received appropriate prophylaxis.[24]

In summary, proper DVT prophylaxis saves lives. There is a substantial reduction in morbidity and duration of hospitalization and

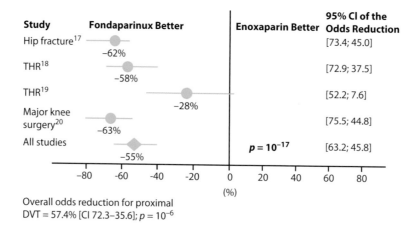

Overall odds reduction for proximal
DVT = 57.4% [CI 72.3–35.6]; $p = 10^{-6}$

Figure 3.2 Graph illustrates odds reduction in patients receiving fondaparinux versus enoxaparin for prophylaxis in orthopedic surgery patients.

rehospitalization, as well as major cost-effectiveness, when appropriate prophylaxis is offered. However, the medical profession has more work to do to ensure that all patients at risk are appropriately protected.

REFERENCES

1. Heit JA, Cohen AT, Anderson FA Jr., et al. Estimated annual number of incident and recurrent, non-fatal and fatal venous thromboembolism (VTE) events in the US. *Blood* 2005; 106:267a.
2. Cohen AT, Agnelli G, Anderson FA, et al. Venous thromboembolism (VTE) in Europe. The number of VTE events and associated morbidity and mortality. *Thromb Haemost* 2007; 98:756–764.
3. Collins R, Scrimgeour A, Yusuf S, et al. Reduction in fatal pulmonary embolism and venous thrombosis by perioperative administration of subcutaneous heparin. Overview of results of randomized trials in general, orthopedic, and urologic surgery. *N Engl J Med* 1988; 318:1162–1173.
4. Heit JA, Silverstein MD, Mohr DN, et al. Risk factors for deep vein thrombosis and pulmonary embolism: a population-based case-control study. *Arch Intern Med* 2000; 160: 809–815.
5. Geerts WH, Pineo GF, Heit JA, et al. Prevention of venous thromboembolism: the Seventh ACCP Conference on Antithrombotic and Thrombolytic Therapy. *Chest* 2004; 126: 338S–400S.
6. Hirsch DR, Ingenito EP, Goldhaber SZ. Prevalence of deep venous thrombosis among patients in medical intensive care. *JAMA* 1995; 274:335–337.
7. Heit JA, O'Fallon WM, Petterson TM, et al. Relative impact of risk factors for deep vein thrombosis and pulmonary embolism: a population-based study. *Arch Intern Med* 2002; 162:1245–1248.
8. Gould MK, Garcia DA, Wren SM, et al. Prevention of VTE in nonorthopedic surgical patients: Antithrombotic Therapy and Prevention of Thrombosis, 9th ed: American College of Chest Physicians Evidence-Based Clinical Practice Guidelines. *Chest* 2012; 141:e227S–e277S.
9. Kahn SR, Lim W, Dunn AS, et al. Prevention of VTE in nonsurgical patients: Antithrombotic Therapy and Prevention of Thrombosis, 9th ed: American College of Chest Physicians Evidence-Based Clinical Practice Guidelines. *Chest* 2012; 141:e195S–e226S.
10. Falck-Ytter Y, Francis CW, Johanson NA, et al. Prevention of VTE in orthopedic surgery patients: Antithrombotic Therapy and Prevention of Thrombosis, 9th ed: American College of Chest Physicians Evidence-Based Clinical Practice Guidelines. *Chest* 2012; 141:e278S–e325S.
11. Dennis M, Sandercock PA, Reid J, et al. Effectiveness of thigh-length graduated compression stockings to reduce the risk of deep vein thrombosis after stroke (CLOTS trial 1): a multicentre, randomised controlled trial. *Lancet* 2009; 373:1958–1965.
12. Malone MD, Cisek PL, Comerota AJ Jr., et al. High-pressure, rapid-inflation pneumatic compression improves venous hemodynamics in healthy volunteers and patients who are post-thrombotic. *J Vasc Surg* 1999; 29:593–599.
13. Comerota AJ, Chouhan V, Harada RN, et al. The fibrinolytic effects of intermittent pneumatic compression: mechanism of enhanced fibrinolysis. *Ann Surg* 1997; 226:306–313.
14. Chouhan VD, Comerota AJ, Sun L, et al. Inhibition of tissue factor pathway during intermittent pneumatic compression: a possible mechanism for antithrombotic effect. *Arterioscler Thromb Vasc Biol* 1999; 19:2812–2817.
15. Eze AR, Cisek PL, Holland BS, et al. The contributions of arterial and venous volumes to increased cutaneous blood flow during leg compression. *Ann Vasc Surg* 1998; 12:182–186.
16. Hull RD, Schellong SM, Tapson VF, et al. Extended-duration venous thromboembolism prophylaxis in acutely ill medical patients with recently reduced mobility: a randomized trial. *Ann Intern Med* 2010; 153:8–18.

17. Bergqvist D, Agnelli G, Cohen AT, et al. Duration of prophylaxis against venous thromboembolism with enoxaparin after surgery for cancer. *N Engl J Med* 2002; 346: 975–980.
18. Wein L, Wein S, Haas SJ, et al. Pharmacological venous thromboembolism prophylaxis in hospitalized medical patients: a meta-analysis of randomized controlled trials. *Arch Intern Med* 2007; 167:1476–1486.
19. Eriksson BI, Bauer KA, Lassen MR, et al. Fondaparinux compared with enoxaparin for the prevention of venous thromboembolism after hip-fracture surgery. *N Engl J Med* 2001; 345:1298–1304.
20. Lassen MR, Bauer KA, Eriksson BI, et al. Postoperative fondaparinux versus preoperative enoxaparin for prevention of venous thromboembolism in elective hip-replacement surgery: a randomised double-blind comparison. *Lancet* 2002; 359:1715–1720.
21. Turpie AG, Bauer KA, Eriksson BI, et al. Postoperative fondaparinux versus postoperative enoxaparin for prevention of venous thromboembolism after elective hip-replacement surgery: a randomised double-blind trial. *Lancet* 2002; 359:1721–1726.
22. Bauer KA, Eriksson BI, Lassen MR, et al. Fondaparinux compared with enoxaparin for the prevention of venous thromboembolism after elective major knee surgery. *N Engl J Med* 2001; 345:1305–1310.
23. Cohen AT, Tapson VF, Bergmann JF, et al. Venous thromboembolism risk and prophylaxis in the acute hospital care setting (ENDORSE study): a multinational cross-sectional study. *Lancet* 2008; 371:387–394.
24. Tapson VF, Decousus H, Pini M, et al. Venous thromboembolism prophylaxis in acutely ill hospitalized medical patients: findings from the International Medical Prevention Registry on Venous Thromboembolism. *Chest* 2007; 132:936–945.

4

Diagnosis of acute DVT

Overview

The clinical diagnosis of acute deep vein thrombosis (DVT) is traditionally regarded as inaccurate and unreliable. In part, this is because the signs and symptoms of acute DVT are confused with the inflammation from infection, pain, and swelling of soft tissue injury, and nonvenous causes of edema. Furthermore, nonocclusive clot may remain asymptomatic until it embolizes, causing signs and symptoms of a pulmonary embolism (PE), or the vein becomes occluded. Therefore, nonocclusive thrombus that does not disturb venous return and which is not associated with inflammation of the vein wall remains asymptomatic. This becomes particularly troublesome when large veins become involved, particularly nonaxial veins such as the hypogastric veins, since pulmonary emboli can occur before leg symptoms, and these emboli can adversely affect cardiopulmonary hemodynamics and potentially result in fatality because of their large size. However, clinical presentation and physical findings can be helpful in patient evaluation.

Clinical evaluation

A careful history and physical examination (H&P) is always helpful. While not achieving the sensitivity, specificity, and predictive value of other objective tests, the H&P should be included in every patient evaluation. The family history, history of cancer, recent trauma, or other pertinent history should be recorded. The physical signs of edema and its location, prominent superficial veins, skin color (hue), tenderness and its location, and the history of spontaneous pain and discomfort and its location are important elements in patient evaluation.

Wells et al.[1] hypothesized that the widely held view that the clinical diagnosis of DVT was unreliable might be incorrect. They developed a clinical model that was prospectively tested in symptomatic outpatients with suspected DVT. They used clinical characteristics (Table 4.1) and assigned them a score. Patients having a score of ≥3 were considered to be at high risk for DVT, those with a score of 0 had a low risk of DVT, and the remaining patients were considered a moderate risk.

In their study of 529 patients, all were clinically assessed to determine the probability of DVT before they underwent definitive diagnostic testing. Results indicated that 85% in the high pretest probability category, 33% in the moderate pretest probability category, and 5% in the low pretest probability category had DVT. These investigators demonstrated that the use of a clinical model when combined with ultrasound would significantly decrease the number of false-positive/negative diagnoses if ascending phlebography was used when the ultrasound result and the pretest probability disagreed. The investigators validated the use of integrating the clinical model as part of the diagnostic strategy for acute DVT.

These authors and others have subsequently integrated D-dimer testing with clinical probability in an effort to conserve vascular laboratory resources and cost of negative ultrasound examinations.

Elf et al.[2] performed a prospective multicenter management study. If a patient was categorized as low pretest probability and the D-dimer

Table 4.1 Pretest clinical probability (Wells' score)

Characteristic	Score
Active cancer	1
Paresis, paralysis, or recent immobilization of lower limb	1
Bedridden > 3 days or major surgery < 4 weeks	1
Localized tenderness	1
Entire leg swollen	1
Calf swelling > 3 cm (compared with asymptomatic limb)	1
Pitting edema	1
Collateral superficial veins	1
Alternative diagnosis as likely or greater than DVT	−2

Source: Data from Wells PS, et al., *Lancet* 1995; 345:1326–1330.

Note: High risk, ≥ 3; moderate risk, 1–2; low risk, 0.

test (moderate sensitivity) was negative, DVT was considered to be ruled out and no further diagnostic test or treatment was offered. In a cohort of 110 patients, only one patient with low pretest probability and negative D-dimer returned within 3 months with an episode of venous thromboembolism (VTE) (0.9%). Others have noted similar results in outpatients with low pretest probability of disease in whom the D-dimer assay was negative.[3] Unfortunately, a negative D-dimer cannot be used to exclude DVT in patients with a high pretest probability, as up to 20% of these patients have subsequently had DVT confirmed.[3]

Ascending phlebography

The recognized gold standard for the objective diagnosis of DVT is ascending contrast phlebography. The technique, which was initially popularized by Rabinov and Paulin,[4] has been refined such that the entire infrainguinal venous system can be well examined through a contrast injection into a pedal vein in the foot. Frequently the iliac veins can be examined from the same injection; however, if more detailed imaging is required, a direct femoral vein puncture is justified.

Contrast opacification of the veins without filling defects excludes DVT (Figure 4.1). An opacified vein with an intraluminal filling defect is diagnostic for DVT (Figure 4.2). Nonfilling of a vein, which occurs with extensive obliteration of the vein by clot, is indirect evidence of DVT (Figure 4.3). Flow voids in veins caused by branch veins carrying nonopacified blood can be responsible for false-positive examination.

Early in its development, ascending phlebography was found to be an accurate test with a high sensitivity and specificity. When compared to postmortem intraosseous phlebography, ascending phlebography was found to have a 97% sensitivity and 95% specificity.[5] Although nonionic contrast has diminished the discomfort of the examination, it remains cumbersome to perform, not all patients have adequate venous access, and there remains the risk of postinjection "phlebitis." Weinmann and Salzman[6] reported a 2% to 3% risk of contrast-induced thrombosis, although the use of nonionic agents, elevation of the leg, and flushing of the contrast with a heparin-saline solution should reduce that risk considerably.

Ascending phlebography remains a useful tool in the diagnostic armamentarium of physicians interested in diagnosing and managing acute DVT; however, in most patients it has largely been supplanted by other techniques, most notably venous duplex ultrasound.

Venous duplex ultrasound

The combination of B-mode imaging with a pulsed Doppler defines *duplex ultrasound*. The pulsed Doppler probe can place the sample volume within the targeted vessel for a specific velocity measurement. Venous duplex ultrasonography is now the diagnostic method of choice for the majority of patients being evaluated for acute DVT. A number of duplex criteria are used in the evaluation of patients for acute DVT (Table 4.2), with the most important being the compressibility of the vein under examination. A normal vein is visible, has a black lumen, and easily compresses with probe pressure (Figure 4.4a,b). Acute thrombus can have the same density as flowing blood with little reflection of soundwaves; therefore, the lumen appears black, similar to a normal vein. However, due

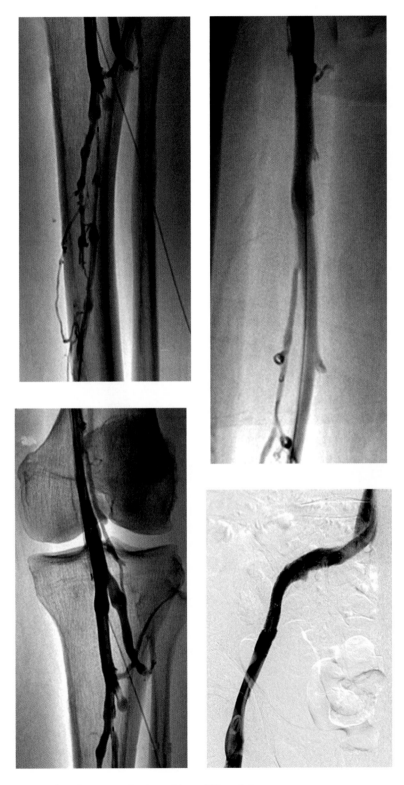

Figure 4.1 Venograms showing normal veins without filling defects.

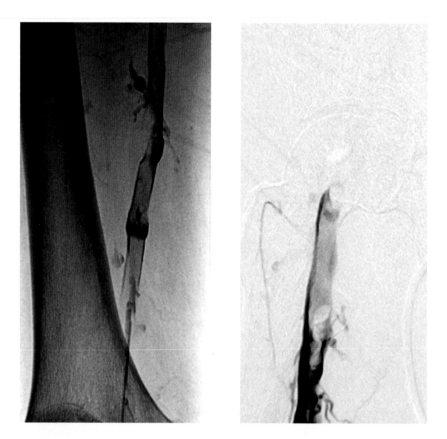

Figure 4.2 Venograms of patient with acute DVT demonstrate filling defect within the femoral vein.

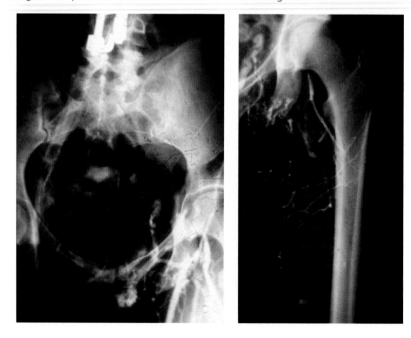

Figure 4.3 Nonvisualization of thrombosed veins is apparent in venograms of a patient with extensive acute DVT.

Table 4.2 Venous duplex diagnosis of acute DVT: Criteria

Component	Criteria
B-mode imaging	Noncompressibility of vein
	Visible intraluminal thrombus
	Dilated veins
	Enlarged branch (tributary) veins (collaterals)
Doppler	Loss of respiratory phasicity
	Loss of spontaneous venous signal
	Abnormal augmentation
	Elevated flow velocity (wind tunnel sound) in main vein
	Elevated flow velocity in branch veins (tributary) (collaterals)

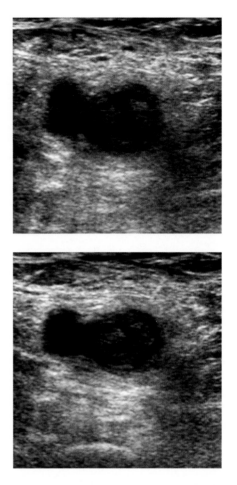

Figure 4.5 Acute clot prevents the vein from being compressed by the Doppler probe.

to the intraluminal thrombus, the vein is non-compressible with probe pressure (Figure 4.5). Noncompressibility is the main criterion for diagnosis in the majority of patients with acute DVT. It should be noted, however, that veins distal to a proximal venous thrombosis, especially distal to iliofemoral venous thrombosis, may have high venous pressures as the result of the proximal occlusion and may be resistant to compression even though no thrombus exists in that vein segment.

As thrombus ages, it may become visible intraluminally (Figure 4.6). Dilated veins and enlarged tributary veins (collaterals) are also visible indicators of acute DVT. The Doppler signal adds valuable information, especially when respiratory phasicity is lost, when spontaneous venous signals cannot be appreciated, and when augmentation (compressing the leg below) is abnormal.

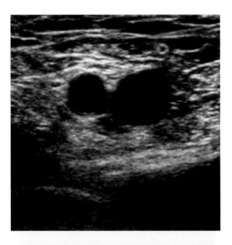

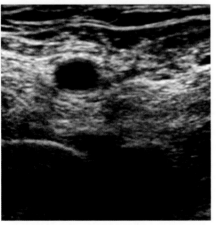

Figure 4.4 Normal vein that is easily compressed by a Doppler probe.

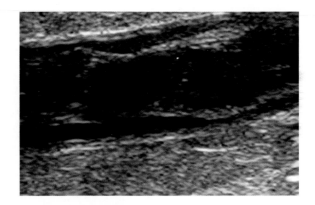

Figure 4.6 Longitudinal view of intraluminal thrombus in a patient with acute DVT.

The venous duplex criteria for diagnosis of acute DVT are listed in Table 4.2. A meta-analysis has shown that noncompressibility is 95% sensitive and 98% specific for proximal DVTs. The specific sensitivities and specificities reported in any single study will depend upon the number of isolated iliac vein and calf vein thromboses included in the patient sample, as these are more difficult to diagnose.

Many investigators and vascular laboratories only perform compression ultrasound of the common femoral and popliteal veins. This limited examination has been adopted to conserve resources and is based on the assumptions that the diagnosis of calf DVT is unreliable, and if calf DVT existed, it would not present serious consequences. However, DVT usually begins in the calf veins[7,8] and isolated calf DVT progresses into the popliteal vein in up to 25% to 30% of patients.[8–11] Pulmonary emboli have been reported in 8% to 34% of patients with isolated calf vein thrombosis.[12] The diagnostic sensitivity and specificity of venous duplex for detecting calf vein thrombosis varies, but investigators interested in this technique have reported sensitivities and specificities up to 90% and 100%, respectively.[13,14] A strategy of a complete ultrasound examination including the calf veins has been compared with limited compression ultrasonography of the proximal veins. Badgett et al.[15] demonstrated that 27% of all abnormal results were the result of calf vein thrombosis. The limited examination would have failed to detect 7.3% of proximal thromboses as well as the 27% of patients with isolated calf vein thrombosis. The complete examination technique added an average of 4 to 5 minutes per extremity.

A negative venous duplex examination reliably excludes DVT, and withholding anticoagulation on the basis of a single (or repeated) negative ultrasound is well established. Noren et al.[16] reported that only 1 of 128 patients (0.8%) with a normal duplex examination returned within 3 months of that negative test with DVT. No patient returned with a PE. Schellong et al.[17] reported a 0.3% thromboembolism rate 3 months after negative results of a complete compression ultrasound. Other investigators have reported similar results when following patients for 3 months without anticoagulation after negative ultrasound.[18]

The negative predictive value of consecutive normal ultrasound examinations has been confirmed by Birdwell et al.[19] and Cogo et al.,[20] where they reported 0.6% and 0.7% DVT event rates within 3 months of two consecutive negative ultrasound examinations.

There is a difference in diagnostic sensitivity of venous ultrasound results when examining symptomatic versus high-risk asymptomatic patients. In a study of postoperative orthopedic patients, 24% of the symptomatic patients and 88% of the asymptomatic patients had isolated calf vein thrombosis.[21] The symptomatic patients had high diagnostic sensitivity and specificity, 85% and 86%, respectively. However, in the asymptomatic group, the sensitivity dropped to 16%, although the specificity was 99%.

Although unusual, isolated iliac vein thrombosis may be difficult to diagnose with venous duplex ultrasound. Clinical suspicion of isolated iliac vein thrombosis occurs when patients have unilateral lower-extremity edema extending from the inguinal ligament distally. Unfortunately, if the thrombus involves the internal iliac vein or is nonocclusive in the common iliac or proximal external iliac vein, it will often remain asymptomatic. The ultrasound criteria for the iliac veins and vena cava differ from those of the infrainguinal vein, as compression of the pelvic veins is generally not possible. Color flow images and venous velocity profiles become more important. Unfortunately, patients who are overweight and those with bowel gas present technical challenges to imaging of the iliac veins, and up to 24% of patients cannot be adequately examined.[22]

Computerized tomographic venography

Computerized tomographic venography (CTV) has many advantages. It can be used with computerized tomographic pulmonary angiography (CTPA) to assess the entire venous system from the calf veins to and including the vena cava after the pulmonary arteries are imaged. One needs to wait 3 to 3.5 minutes after the injection of the contrast used for CTPA to begin imaging the lower-extremity venous system. The major disadvantage of CTV is the radiation exposure, which can be considerable when a full pulmonary arteriogram and CTV are performed.[23] Although an attractive option for imaging, it is infrequently used. Perhaps its major advantage is the imaging of pelvic veins in patients considered at risk of pelvic DVT.

One of the inherent advantages of both types of cross-sectional imaging (CTV and magnetic resonance venography [MRV]) is the capability of showing additional abdominal, pelvic, and chest pathology that may be etiologically associated with the development of venous thrombosis, such as pelvic masses or abdominal or thoracic malignancies (Figure 4.7a–c). One can also show iliac vein compression as a result of an overlying artery.

Magnetic resonance venography

MRV is slowly increasing in popularity. With the improvements in imaging, it is now an option in some patients who may be difficult to diagnose, particularly those with pelvic venous thrombosis. A number of MRV techniques are used, including spin echo, gradient, recalled echo, and the use of intravenous gadolinium. Similar to ascending phlebography, the absence of an image or a flow void (a filling defect) within a visible vein suggests the presence of thrombus. However, there are well-known flow artifacts that can often produce a false-positive image. With computerized manipulation, the images can be rotated such that multiple axial, coronal, and sagittal planes are available for examination following skilled postprocessing.

In a prospective blinded study, MRV was found to have excellent accuracy. A sensitivity of 97% and specificity of 100% were reported by Fraser and Anderson[13] with very little interobserver variability.

Unfortunately, MRV continues to be expensive, is often not available, some patients are claustrophobic, and it is not a friendly technique for follow-up examinations.

D-dimer tests

The use of a blood test to establish whether a patient has DVT or, stated more precisely, to rule out DVT has become increasingly popular, as noted earlier in this chapter. D-dimer is a sensitive test measuring breakdown of complexed fibrin. The family of D-dimers represents breakdown products of cross-linked fibrin that have been stabilized by factor XIII.[24] When plasmin breaks down complexed fibrin, D-dimer is released. Thus, the presence of D-dimer is an indicator of blood clot, although its location, clinical importance, and other important details are absent. Many conditions, such as inflammation, recent surgery, infection, and pregnancy, produce elevated D-dimers.

A negative test is helpful in excluding DVT, whereas a positive test is frequently not helpful, as discussed earlier. Wells et al.[1,25] and others[2] have shown that the combination of a low clinical suspicion and a negative D-dimer results in a 99% negative predictive value for DVT. In this scenario, no further testing is required and anticoagulation can be safely withheld.

The prospective and large retrospective studies using clinical assessment to gauge pretest probability of DVT supplemented by D-dimer and venous duplex have illustrated how these can be used for the accurate evaluation of patients with suspected DVT. Figure 4.8 is a suggested

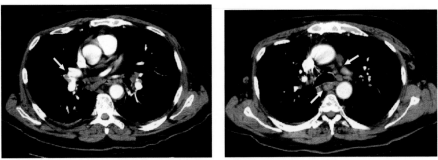

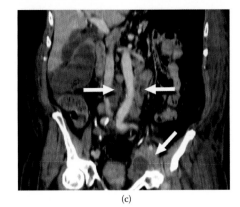

Figure 4.7 (a) CT scan of chest with contrast in a patient with iliofemoral DVT shows bilateral asymptomatic pulmonary emboli (arrow). (b) Additional images of chest show enlarged mediastinal lymph nodes (arrows) compressing the trachea. (c) CT scan of the abdomen shows enlarged retroperitoneal and pelvic lymph nodes (arrows) due to an undiagnosed lymphoma.

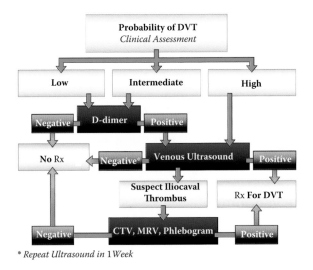

Figure 4.8 Suggested diagnostic strategy for patients suspected of having acute DVT.

algorithm for the assessment of patients with suspected DVT.

REFERENCES

1. Wells PS, Hirsh J, Anderson DR, et al. Accuracy of clinical assessment of deep-vein thrombosis. *Lancet* 1995; 345:1326–1330.
2. Elf JL, Strandberg K, Nilsson C, Svensson PJ. Clinical probability assessment and D-dimer determination in patients with suspected deep vein thrombosis, a prospective multicenter management study. *Thromb Res* 2009; 123:612–616.
3. Kelly J, Hunt BJ. Role of D-dimers in diagnosis of venous thromboembolism. *Lancet* 2002; 359:456–458.
4. Rabinov K, Paulin S. Roentgen diagnosis of venous thrombosis in the leg. *Arch Surg* 1972; 104:134–144.
5. Lund F, Diener L, Ericsson JL. Postmortem intraosseous phlebography as an aid in studies of venous thromboembolism. With application on a geriatric clientele. *Angiology* 1969; 20:155–176.
6. Weinmann EE, Salzman EW. Deep-vein thrombosis. *N Engl J Med* 1994; 331: 1630–1641.
7. Cogo A, Lensing AW, Prandoni P, Hirsh J. Distribution of thrombosis in patients with symptomatic deep vein thrombosis. Implications for simplifying the diagnostic process with compression ultrasound. *Arch Intern Med* 1993; 153:2777–2780.
8. Philbrick JT, Becker DM. Calf deep venous thrombosis. A wolf in sheep's clothing? *Arch Intern Med* 1988; 148:2131–2138.
9. Lagerstedt CI, Olsson CG, Fagher BO, Oqvist BW, Albrechtsson U. Need for long-term anticoagulant treatment in symptomatic calf-vein thrombosis. *Lancet* 1985; 2: 515–518.
10. Huisman MV, Buller HR, ten Cate JW, Vreeken J. Serial impedance plethysmography for suspected deep venous thrombosis in outpatients. The Amsterdam General Practitioner Study. *N Engl J Med* 1986; 314:823–828.
11. Lohr JM, James KV, Deshmukh RM, Hasselfeld KA, Allastair B. Karmody Award. Calf vein thrombi are not a benign finding. *Am J Surg* 1995; 170:86–90.
12. Moreno-Cabral R, Kistner RL, Nordyke RA. Importance of calf vein thrombophlebitis. *Surgery* 1976; 80:735–742.
13. Fraser JD, Anderson DR. Deep venous thrombosis: recent advances and optimal investigation with US. *Radiology* 1999; 211:9–24.
14. Elias A, Le CG, Bouvier JL, Benichou M, Serradimigni A. Value of real time B mode ultrasound imaging in the diagnosis of deep vein thrombosis of the lower limbs. *Int Angiol* 1987; 6:175–182.
15. Badgett DK, Comerota MC, Khan MN, Eid IG, Kerr RP, Comerota AJ. Duplex venous imaging: role for a comprehensive lower extremity examination. *Ann Vasc Surg* 2000; 14:73–76.
16. Noren A, Lindmarker P, Rosfors S. A retrospective follow-up study of patients with suspected deep vein thrombosis and negative results of colour duplex ultrasound. *Phlebography* 1997; 12:56–59.
17. Schellong SM, Schwarz T, Halbritter K, et al. Complete compression ultrasonography of the leg veins as a single test for the diagnosis of deep vein thrombosis. *Thromb Haemost* 2003; 89:228–234.
18. Elias A, Mallard L, Elias M, et al. A single complete ultrasound investigation of the venous network for the diagnostic management of patients with a clinically suspected first episode of deep venous thrombosis of the lower limbs. *Thromb Haemost* 2003; 89:221–227.
19. Birdwell BG, Raskob GE, Whitsett TL, et al. The clinical validity of normal compression ultrasonography in outpatients suspected of having deep venous thrombosis. *Ann Intern Med* 1998; 128:1–7.
20. Cogo A, Lensing AW, Koopman MM, et al. Compression ultrasonography for diagnostic management of patients with clinically suspected deep vein thrombosis: prospective cohort study. *BMJ* 1998; 316: 17–20.

21. Sumner DS. Diagnosis of deep vein thrombosis with real-time color and duplex scanning. In Bernstein EF (ed.), *Vascular diagnosis*. St. Louis: Mosby, 1993: 794–795.

22. Messina LM, Sarpa MS, Smith MA, Greenfield LJ. Clinical significance of routine imaging of iliac and calf veins by color flow duplex scanning in patients suspected of having acute lower extremity deep venous thrombosis. *Surgery* 1993; 114:921–927.

23. Katz DS, Hon M. Current DVT imaging. *Tech Vasc Interv Radiol* 2004; 7:55–62.

24. Bauer KA. Laboratory markers of coagulation and fibrinolysis. In Colman RW, Marder VJ, Clowes A, Genge JN, Goldhaber SZ (eds.), *Hemostasis and thrombosis*. Philadelphia: Lippincott, Williams & Wilkins, 2006: 835–850.

25. Wells PS. Integrated strategies for the diagnosis of venous thromboembolism. *J Thromb Haemost* 2007; 5(Suppl 1):41–50.

5

Anticoagulants

Overview

Anticoagulation with unfractionated heparin (UFH) followed by oral vitamin K antagonists (VKAs) has been the mainstay of therapy for acute deep vein thrombosis (DVT). For 50 years, the recognition and refinement of the mechanisms of action of heparin led to the discovery of low-molecular-weight heparin (LMWH) compounds and subsequently the pentasaccharide fondaparinux. A new generation of anticoagulants, oral direct factor Xa inhibitors, are becoming available and are discussed separately in Chapter 6.

Anticoagulation is essentially a prophylactic, since these agents interrupt thrombus formation but do not actively dissolve thrombus. However, effective anticoagulation prevents clot formation and protects the body's endogenous fibrinolytic system, and offers the opportunity to reduce the thrombus burden and recanalize the occluded vein.

Unfractionated heparin

Since its discovery in 1916 by McLean,[1] heparin was established as an effective anticoagulant. It is the drug most frequently used by vascular surgeons during interventional and operative procedures, and is used for venous thromboembolism (VTE) prophylaxis and treatment for patients with cardiac and arterial vascular thrombotic disorders. To achieve its anticoagulant effect, heparin binds to antithrombin III, producing a conformational change that converts antithrombin III from a slow to a rapid inhibitor of fibrin.[2] Preparations of heparin in clinical use contain molecular weights ranging from 3,000 to 30,000 Daltons, and less than one-half of the administered heparin is responsible for the anticoagulation effect by binding to the antithrombin III molecule.[3,4] A secondary anticoagulation effect is achieved through binding with heparin cofactor II,[5] although higher doses of heparin must be administered than those usually given. Heparin has other effects independent of its anticoagulant activity that may play an important role in the patient's overall antithrombotic status. Heparin inhibits platelet function and prolongs bleeding time,[6,7] and it inhibits vascular smooth muscle cells and binds to vascular endothelium.[8,9] These secondary effects may become particularly important after invasive procedures such as angiography, cardiac catheterization, and angioplasty, both by improving results and by increasing complications.

The heparin–antithrombin III complex inactivates thrombin (factor IIa) and activated clotting factors IX, X, XI, and XII. Evidence is increasing that heparin's inhibitory effect on anticoagulation is mediated through the inhibition of thrombin-induced activation of factors V and VIII (Figure 5.1).[10–12]

When used clinically, heparin does not follow simple first-order kinetics. When higher doses of heparin are given, a longer disappearance time and decreased clearance are observed; therefore, the dose-response relationship is not linear. The anticoagulant response increases disproportionately as the dose increases.[13–16]

Heparin's action may be prevented by platelets, fibrin, and circulating plasma proteins.

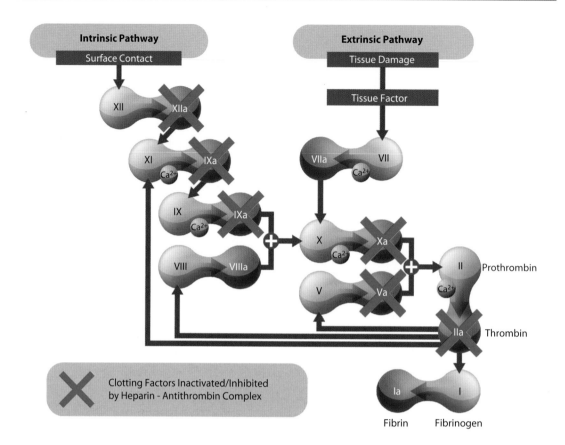

Figure 5.1 Illustration shows clotting factors affected by the heparin–antithrombin complex.

Platelets secrete platelet factor IV,[17] which actively neutralizes the anticoagulant activity of heparin. Two other plasma proteins, histidine-rich glycoprotein[18] and vitronectin,[19] also neutralize the anticoagulant effect of heparin. Additionally, when factor Xa is bound to platelets, the anticoagulant effect of the heparin–antithrombin III complex is ineffective. The effect of heparin's interaction on the plasminogen-plasmin enzyme system has been studied, and heparin has been found to enhance the activation of circulating plasminogen to plasmin, but it paradoxically impairs the activation of the fibrin-bound plasminogen. The net overall effect of heparin on endovenous fibrinolytic activity is small, and it most likely neither enhances nor inhibits endogenous fibrinolysis.[20,21]

Heparin is poorly absorbed through the gastrointestinal tract or intrabronchially; therefore, it must be given parenterally for reliable therapy. Heparin is effective after subcutaneous injection and when given intravenously. The anticoagulant response to heparin in any individual is unpredictable, and monitoring of the activated partial thromboplastin time (aPTT) is therefore necessary to ensure the desired therapeutic response.

Heparin induces antihemostatic effects through three mechanisms: (1) it binds to antithrombin III and inactivates factors IIa, Xa, XIa, and XIIa; (2) it binds to cofactor II and inactivates factor IIa; and (3) it binds to factor IX and inhibits factor Xa activation. The major mechanism for the anticoagulation effect is through antithrombin III.

The two routes for administration of UFH are continuous infusion and subcutaneous injection. Heparin is cleared through a combination of saturable cellular mechanisms and a slower, first-order, nonsaturable, dose-dependent mechanism of renal clearance. At therapeutic doses, heparin is cleared through the rapid, saturable, dose-dependent mechanism. These pharmacokinetics make the heparin anticoagulation response nonlinear at therapeutic doses, with both the intensity and duration of effect increasing disproportionately at increasing dose. The initial dose of heparin for treatment of DVT is weight based (80 U/kg bolus followed by 18 U/kg/hr continuous infusion). The anticoagulant effect of heparin is monitored by the aPTT when the usual therapeutic dose is used. An aPTT of 1.5 to 2.5 times the control value was shown to be associated with a decreased risk of recurrent VTE. The aPTT should be measured no earlier than 6 hours after the bolus dose, and the continuous infusion should be adjusted accordingly.

It is commonly believed that the risk of bleeding with UFH increases as the dose increases, and that patients with increased risk can be identified by *in vitro* coagulation tests used to monitor heparin therapy. There may be some merit to this observation in patients who have comorbid risk factors that identify patients at high risk.[22] However, in patients without comorbid risk factors, whether a therapeutic or supratherapeutic aPTT is targeted does not appear to be related to an increased risk of clinically important bleeding complications.[23] Even though the importance of maintaining therapeutic anticoagulation from the initiation of therapy has been established,[24] audits of heparin anticoagulation indicate that a large number of patients continue to be inadequately treated,[25] and that after a subtherapeutic aPTT was found, no alteration in heparin infusion was ordered in 33% of patients. Investigators have confirmed that a prescriptive approach to heparin administration is more effective than the subjective, individual approach attempted by most clinicians.[26,27] This assumes substantial clinical importance when one considers that a subtherapeutic aPTT (<1.5 × control) early in the course of treatment is associated with a 15-fold risk of recurrence.

In order to avoid undertreatment, supratherapeutic heparin anticoagulation during the initial 4 to 5 days of therapy can be offered to patients who do not have comorbidities for bleeding.[23] A 10,000 IU heparin bolus is given intravenously and followed by 2000 IU per hour, checking the aPTT 8 hours following the bolus. The goal is to maintain the aPTT greater than 90 seconds. If the aPTT is supratherapeutic (>100 seconds), the dose is continued. While this approach varies from most protocols, it has been effective in maintaining therapeutic anticoagulation without added bleeding in patients without associated comorbidities. Using the prescriptive approach summarized in Table 5.1 is a good option and favored by most physicians. However, even with the prescriptive approach, one must be cautious in patients with comorbidities for bleeding.

Heparin resistance is a term used to define patients who need unusually large doses of heparin to achieve an anticoagulation effect. Several mechanisms have been identified for heparin resistance,

Table 5.1 Prescriptive approach to intravenous heparin therapy

	Intravenous infusion		
aPTT[a]	Rate change (mL/h)	Dose change (units 24 h)[b]	Additional action
≤45	+6	+5760	Repeat aPTT in 4–6 hours
46–54	+3	+2880	Repeat aPTT in 4–6 hours
55–85	0	0	None[c]
86–110	−3	−2880	Stop heparin sodium treatment for 1 hour; repeat aPTT 4–6 hours after restarting heparin treatment
>110	−6	−5760	Stop heparin sodium treatment for 1 hour; repeat aPTT 4–6 hours after restarting heparin treatment

[a] Activated partial thromboplastin time.

[b] Heparin sodium concentration, 20,000 units/500 mL = 40 units/mL.

[c] During the first 24 hours, repeat aPTT in 4–6 hours. Thereafter, the aPTT will be determined once daily, unless subtherapeutic.

including ATIII deficiency, increased heparin clearance, elevations in heparin-binding proteins, high factor VII, and fibrinogen levels. A large thrombus burden also requires higher heparin concentrations for therapeutic effectiveness. Randomized trials have shown that oral anticoagulation alone, without initial and concomitant heparin anticoagulation, is associated with a significantly higher risk of recurrent venous thrombosis.[28]

Low-molecular-weight heparins

LMWHs are derived from UFH through chemical or enzymatic depolymerization. The LMWHs have several advantages compared to UFH, including (1) a reduced antifactor IIA activity relative to Xa activity, (2) greater benefit/risk ratio in animal studies, (3) superior pharmacokinetic properties (improved bioavailability when injected subcutaneously), (4) no need for monitoring (possible exceptions being pregnancy and morbid obesity), and (5) less risk of heparin-induced thrombocytopenia (HIT). Compared with UFH, LMWHs have a longer plasmin half-life (approximately 4.5 hours) and substantially higher plasma levels after subcutaneous injection. Bioavailability studies have demonstrated that 90% of LMWHs injected subcutaneously can be retrieved from the blood.[29,30] As a result of the improved bioavailability, they have less variability in anticoagulant response following a fixed dose. The reduced binding to plasma proteins is responsible for the more predictable dose-response relationship of LMWHs.

LMWHs are approved for DVT prophylaxis in general surgical and orthopedic patients, for the treatment of acute DVT and pulmonary embolism (PE), and for the prevention of ischemic complications of unstable angina and non-Q-wave myocardial infarction. The evidence that LMWHs are safe and effective for the treatment of acute DVT is impressive. Randomized trials comparing LMWH with UFH for VTE prophylaxis and treatment of established VTE have demonstrated the advantage of LMWH. Treatment trials have shown better thrombus resolution and fewer bleeding complications with LMWH.[31,32] In two trials, mortality was significantly reduced in those randomized to LMWH; however, the survival benefit of LWMH appeared limited to patients with malignancy.

Long-term LMWH has been compared with VKAs in patients with proximal DVT.[31] It appears that LMWH is a valuable alternative to VKAs, particularly in patients who have recurrent DVT or PE while on therapeutic doses of warfarin. Long-term LMWH has also been compared with VKAs in patients with cancer and proximal DVT.[32,33] Results demonstrated a reduction in recurrence of VTE and fewer bleeding complications with LMWH.

In the pregnant and morbidly obese patient being treated for acute DVT with LMWH, monitoring of the mid-interval Xa level has been suggested to ensure therapeutic anticoagulation. The target Xa level depends upon the frequency of dosing. A target Xa level of 0.6 to 1.0 for 12-hour dosing and 0.8 to 1.5 for 24-hour dosing is recommended.

Fondaparinux

Fondaparinux is a small synthetic pentasaccharide (mw 1728) that is an indirect factor Xa inhibitor. Fondaparinux binds to antithrombin, thereby changing its binding site and allowing it to neutralize factor Xa.[34] Once fondaparinux binds to antithrombin, it produces a conformational change increasing antithrombin's ability to bind factor Xa, resulting in a 300-fold increase in the rate of factor Xa inhibition by antithrombin. Once Xa is bound to the fondaparinux–antithrombin complex, fondaparinux is released, permitting the same molecule of fondaparinux to recycle and bind to another molecule of antithrombin (Figure 5.2). Since the pentasaccharide is a small molecule, it does not bridge antithrombin to thrombin; therefore, fondaparinux does not inhibit thrombin.

Fondaparinux has no significant protein binding, has excellent bioavailability following subcutaneous injection, and has a plasma half-life of 17 to 20 hours. Similar to LMWHs, fondaparinux is excreted through the kidneys. As a result, it is generally recommended that fondaparinux not be used in those with renal insufficiency, and if it is, dose adjustment is necessary. Because fondaparinux does not bind to platelets or platelet factor IV, there is no resulting antibody production that might cause HIT. In the entire experience with fondaparinux, only one case of HIT has been reported.[35]

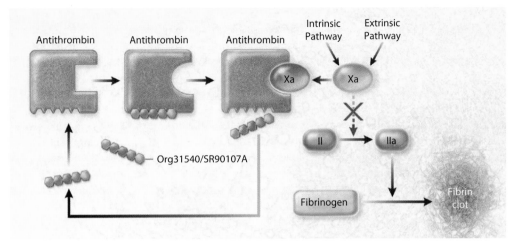

Figure 5.2 The red X indicates that the inhibition of activated factor X leads to interruption of the coagulation cascade by preventing the activation of factor II (prothrombin) to factor IIa (thrombin). Org31540/SR90107A binds with high affinity to the pentasaccharide binding site on antithrombin, producing an irreversible conformational change in antithrombin; an arginine residue is exposed, which binds to and inhibits activated factor X, a key factor in the activation of coagulation. Org31540/SR90107A is then released and made available to bind to other antithrombin molecules. (From Turpie AG, et al., *N Engl J Med* 2001; 344:619–625.[36] With permission.)

Fondaparinux is a synthetic molecule that has a high affinity for antithrombin. It has approximately a sevenfold increase in anti-Xa activity compared with LMWH.

Fondaparinux is used at a dose of 2.5 mg for prophylaxis of VTE and is given at a dose of 7.5 mg for treatment of VTE in patients weighing 50 to 100 kg. Because of its excellent bioavailability, it can be used in a once-a-day dose regimen. The dose is decreased to 5 mg for patients weighing less than 50 kg and increased to 10 mg for those weighing more than 100 kg. Fondaparinux has been used to prevent thrombotic complications of acute coronary syndromes at a dose of 2.5 mg daily.

There is no known antidote to fondaparinux, and it is not bound by a protamine sulfate. In patients who develop bleeding complications after fondaparinux has been given, recombinant factor VIIa may be helpful.

Direct thrombin inhibitors

Thrombin can be inhibited directly or indirectly. Direct inhibitors bind to the thrombin molecule, blocking its interaction with other substrates and reducing additional thrombus formation. Indirect inhibitors (i.e., heparin) act by catalyzing antithrombin or heparin cofactor II. In the growing population of patients with HIT, direct thrombin inhibitors offer valuable therapeutic alternatives. Three intravenous direct thrombin inhibitors (lepirudin, argatroban, and bivalirudin) have been licensed in North America.

Lepirudin

Lepirudin is a recombinant hirudin. It is a 65-amino acid polypeptide that was originally isolated from the salivary glands of the leach *Hirudo medicinalis*. Lepirudin irreversibly binds to thrombin, which is one of its potential disadvantages since there is no specific antidote. The plasma half-life is approximately 60 minutes after IV injection. It is cleared by the kidneys and therefore must be used with caution in anyone with compromised renal function. The anticoagulant effect can be monitored by the aPTT. Lepirudin is indicated for anticoagulation in patients with HIT and associated thromboembolic disease to prevent further thromboembolic complications. Lepirudin is particularly useful in patients with HIT associated with hepatic dysfunction, since argatroban is contraindicated in these patients. As with other anticoagulants, bleeding is the most common adverse side effect. Serious anaphylactic reactions have been reported.

Greinacher et al.[37] conducted two prospective, multicenter, historically controlled trials in 113 patients with confirmed HIT. It was observed that by day 35 in the HIT-1 study, the group treated with lepirudin showed a relative reduction of the cumulative risk for combined clinical endpoints (death, limb amputation, new thromboembolic complications) by 73% versus historical controls. The same author published a meta-analysis of the HIT-1 and HIT-2 studies, confirming a statistically significant difference in the combined incidence of death, new thromboembolic complications, and amputations in patients treated with lepirudin versus historical controls in the subgroup of patients with thromboembolic complications from HIT. Relative risks for individual events also decreased.

When starting lepirudin, an initial aPTT is obtained. If >2.4, lepirudin is held to avoid initial overdosing. When treating a patient with thrombosis and HIT, an initial dose (bolus) of 0.4 mg/kg over 15 to 20 seconds is given followed by continuous infusion of 0.10 mg/kg/hr. The duration of therapy is 5 to 10 days and generally depends upon the indication for initial anticoagulation. If the patient is not being treated for established thrombosis, the initial bolus dose is withheld.

Argatroban

Argatroban is a competitive inhibitor of thrombin that binds noncovalently to form a reversible complex. Its half-life is 45 minutes. Since argatroban is metabolized in the liver, it must be used with caution in patients with compromised hepatic function. Argatroban nearly meets the requirements of the ideal anticoagulant for both the prophylaxis and treatment of HIT and associated thrombotic complications. As the first direct thrombin inhibitor approved for both prophylaxis and treatment of thrombosis in HIT, argatroban is an effective anticoagulant that does not interact with heparin-dependent antibodies, offers a predictable dose-response relationship, and requires minimal monitoring. Therefore, it is frequently chosen to manage patients with HIT.

Before initiating argatroban, heparin is discontinued, allowing the aPTT to return to baseline. The initial dose of argatroban for adults without hepatic impairment is 2 mg/kg/min administered in a continuous intravenous infusion.[38,39] The aPTT should be rechecked 2 hours after initiation, and the dose should be adjusted until the target aPTT value of 1.5 to 3.0 times baseline is obtained (not to exceed 100 sec). Concomitant use of argatroban with warfarin results in prolongation of the international normalized ratio (INR) beyond that produced by warfarin alone. When patients are being converted to vitamin K antagonists, at least 4 days of overlap is given. After this period, argatroban can be discontinued when the INR is greater than 4. After stopping argatroban, a repeat INR is obtained in 4 to 6 hours. If the repeat INR is below the desired therapeutic range, infusion of argatroban is resumed and the procedure repeated on a daily basis until the desired INR is achieved with warfarin alone.

Bivalirudin

Bivalirudin is an analog of lepirudin that reversibly binds to the active form of thrombin. Once bound, thrombin cleaves the bond within the amino terminal of bivalirudin, allowing the recovery of thrombin activity and making it a potentially safer drug than lepirudin. Bivalirudin is cleared from plasma by a combination of renal mechanisms and proteolytic cleavage, having a half-life in patients with normal renal function of approximately 25 minutes. It is a convenient drug to use because of its short half-life and its predictable anticoagulation response in patients undergoing percutaneous coronary interventions.[40–42]

The recommended dose of bivalirudin is an initial bolus of 1 mg/kg intravenously followed by a 4-hour intravenous infusion rate of 2.5 mg/kg/hr. If necessary, bivalirudin may be continued for an additional 20 hours at a rate of 0.2/mg/kg/hr, adjusting the dose to keep the aPTT at 1.5 to 2.5 × baseline. Bivalirudin is predominantly used as an alternative to heparin during percutaneous endovascular procedures. Additional uses of this compound are currently being investigated, including its use as effective treatment for patients with HIT.

Warfarin compounds (Vitamin K antagonists)

Oral anticoagulation with VKAs produces their anticoagulant effect by inhibiting the vitamin K-dependent coagulation factors II, VII, IX, and X.[43,44] Oral anticoagulants also inhibit vitamin K-dependent carboxylation of proteins C and S. Because proteins C and S are naturally occurring anticoagulants that function by inhibiting activated factors V and VIII, VKAs produce a procoagulant state before they achieve their anticoagulant effect due to the half-lives of proteins C and S being much shorter than the half-lives of the clotting factors. The warfarin compounds do not have an immediate effect on the coagulation system because the existing coagulation factors in the circulation must be cleared. Generally, warfarin compounds must be administered for 4 to 5 days to achieve therapeutic anticoagulation. The peak effect of a VKA does not occur until 36 to 72 hours after drug administration.[45–47] During the first several days of treatment with warfarin, the prothrombin time reflects the change in factor VII level, which has a short half-life of 5 to 7 hours. Effective depression of the levels of clotting factors II, IX, and X is not reached until 5 to 7 days after the VKA is started.[46–48] Therefore, patients should be treated during this time with either intravenous UFH or subcutaneous LMWH. As previously mentioned, primary therapy with VKAs without heparin therapy is associated with unacceptably high recurrent thromboembolic complications.[28]

In clinical practice, VKAs require careful monitoring for a number of reasons: (1) they have a narrow therapeutic window; (2) they have variability in dose effect among subjects; (3) their activity is influenced by a large number of drugs and diet; and (4) miscommunication between physician and patient and noncompliance of the patient substantially impact the outcome.

Evidence indicates that the anticoagulant and antithrombotic effects of VKAs can be disassociated, and that the reduction of factors II and X is required for effective anticoagulation. Studies have shown that warfarin produces its thrombotic effect by reducing factor II levels, which is consistent with observations that clot-bound thrombin is an important mediator of clot growth and reduction in prothrombin levels reduces the generation of thrombin, thereby reducing thrombus formation. This is the pharmacologic basis for overlapping the administration of heparin with warfarin for at least 4 to 5 days and until the prothrombin time/INR is therapeutic. Since the half-life of factor II is approximately 60 to 72 hours, at least 4 to 5 days of overlap is necessary to ensure a proper anticoagulant effect, even if the INR reaches therapeutic levels sooner. The prothrombin time (PT) test is the proper test to monitor VKA therapy. The PT reflects the reduction of three of the four vitamin K-dependent factors that are affected by warfarin compounds. Several randomized studies have compared an INR of 2.0 to 3.0 to a higher-intensity adjusted dose. An INR of 2.0 to 3.0 gave the best antithrombotic effect at the lowest risk of bleeding. Recommendations for the initiation of oral anticoagulation suggest that a dose between 5 and 10 mg for the first 1 to 2 days, followed by dosing according to the INR response, is the most appropriate. Monitoring this is performed daily, starting after the second or third dose until the therapeutic range is achieved and maintained for at least 2 days before heparin is discontinued.

The management of patients whose INR is outside the therapeutic range is controversial due to the lack of comparison studies. Our approach is to monitor more frequently and adjust the dose appropriately or, if the INR is higher than 4.0, hold warfarin for a period of time and monitor more frequently to adjust the dose (Table 5.2). Treatment directed at reversing the anticoagulant effect with VKAs, fresh frozen plasma, or recombinant factor VIIa is based on clinical judgment and a proscribed protocol.

Warfarin compounds cross the placenta and have been associated with teratogenic effects when given during the first trimester of pregnancy. Because there are similar concerns in the second trimester as well as the risk of fetal bleeding during and after delivery, warfarin compounds are avoided when treating pregnant women. Women who are of childbearing potential and taking warfarin compounds should avoid pregnancy and receive contraceptive counseling. If anticoagulation is indicated during pregnancy, subcutaneous LMWH is the anticoagulant of choice.

Table 5.2 Anticoagulation dosing algorithm for INR range 2.0–3.0

INR	Action
<1.5	Increase weekly dose by 10–15%, repeat INR in 4–7 days. Consider extra dose.
	Notify physician if <1.5 × 2 INRs for evaluation and need for UFH, LMWH.
1.51–1.79	Increase weekly dose by 5–10%, repeat INR in 7–10 days.
1.80–1.99	No change. Repeat INR in 7–10 days.
2.0–3.0	No change. Repeat INR based on follow-up algorithm.
3.01–3.30	No change. Repeat INR in 7–14 days.
3.31–3.49	Decrease dosing by 5%, repeat INR in 7–10 days.
3.5–3.99	Decrease weekly dose by 5–10%, repeat INR in 7–10 days.
4.0–4.99	Hold 1 dose of warfarin and repeat INR next day, decrease weekly dose by 10%, repeat INR in 4–7 days.
5.0–5.99 No significant bleeding	Omit 1–2 doses, repeat INR next day to be sure INR is decreasing, decrease weekly dose by 10–15%, and repeat INR in 4–7 days. Assess for bleeding and risk factors.
6.0–8.99 No significant bleeding	Hold next dose and check INR next day to insure INR is decreasing. Hold next 2 doses and repeat INR on third day. Resume at lower dose when INR in therapeutic range, decreasing weekly dose by 15%. Assess for bleeding and risk factors; alternatively, consider giving vitamin K 1.0–2.5 mg p.o. if at increased risk for bleeding.
	Notify physician of INR. Physician order must be obtained for vitamin K administration.
>9.0 No significant bleeding	Omit warfarin, assess for bleeding and risk factors. Consider vitamin K 2.5–5.0 mg p.o., monitor INR daily, resume at lower dose when INR in therapeutic range decreasing weekly dose by 15–20%.
	Notify physician of INR. Physician order must be obtained for vitamin K administration.
Serious bleeding at any elevation of INR	Omit warfarin, **contact physician** (consider vitamin K 5.0–10 mg IV slow infusion, supplemented with fresh frozen plasma depending on the urgency of the situation; vitamin K can be repeated every 12 hours). Physician order must be obtained for vitamin K administration.

Note: Always consider trend in INRs when making warfarin management decisions. Consider repeating INR same day or next day if observed INR is markedly different than expected value. Potential for lab errors exists.

Follow-Up Algorithm

Consecutive days in range (INR)	Recheck INR in
1–10	1 week
11–14	2 weeks
15–21	3 weeks
22–30	4 weeks

Note: If INR 2.0–2.1 or 2.9–3.0, repeat INR in 2 weeks regardless of the number of consecutive in-range INRs. For patients with many consecutive therapeutic INRs, the follow-up algorithm may be accelerated by the protime nurse for a single out-of-range INR.

Danaparoid

Danaparoid is considered a heparinoid, a mixture of glycosaminoglycans composed of heperan sulfate, dermatan sulfate, and chondroitin sulfate, which functions through antithrombin-dependent inhibition of factor Xa. Its half-life is 18 to 24 hours and it is renally excreted. Danaparoid is unique in that it suppresses HIT antibody-induced platelet aggregation, a property not observed with other pharmacologic agents used for the treatment of HIT.[49] The anticoagulant activity of danaparoid is monitored by measuring antifactor Xa activity, although this is generally not required, as there is a predictable response when administered on a weight basis. There is no antidote to danaparoid. Danaparoid was removed from the market in the United States, presumably due to a low cross-reactivity rate with HIT antibodies, although this rarely has clinical consequences. Danaparoid is commonly used in Europe, Canada, Australia, and New Zealand.

Danaparoid is administered intravenously with a bolus of 2250 units followed by an infusion of 400 U/hr for 4 hours, 300 U/hr for 4 hours, and then 200 U/hr for at least 5 days or longer. Interestingly, among all of the pharmacologic agents used for the treatment of HIT, danaparoid is the only agent whose outcome has been evaluated in a prospective, randomized, controlled study.[50]

REFERENCES

1. McLean J. The thromboplastic action of cephalin. *Am J Physiol* 1916; 41:250.
2. Rosenberg RD. The heparin-antithrombin system: a natural anticoagulation mechanism. In Colman RW, Hirsh J, Marder VJ, Salzman EW (eds.), *Hemostasis and thrombosis*. Philadelphia: JB Lippincott, 1987: 1373–1392.
3. Lam LH, Silbert JE, Rosenberg RD. The separation of active and inactive forms of heparin. *Biochem Biophys Res Commun* 1976; 69:570–577.
4. Andersson LO, Barrowcliffe TW, Holmer E, Johnson EA, Sims GE. Anticoagulant properties of heparin fractionated by affinity chromatography on matrix-bound antithrombin III and by gel filtration. *Thromb Res* 1976; 9:575–583.
5. Ofosu FA, Modi GJ, Hirsh J, Buchanan MR, Blajchman MA. Mechanisms for inhibition of the generation of thrombin activity by sulfated polysaccharides. *Ann N Y Acad Sci* 1986; 485:41–55.
6. Castellot JJ Jr., Favreau LV, Karnovsky MJ, Rosenberg RD. Inhibition of vascular smooth muscle cell growth by endothelial cell-derived heparin. Possible role of a platelet endoglycosidase. *J Biol Chem* 1982; 257:11256–11260.
7. Heiden D, Mielke CH Jr., Rodvien R. Impairment by heparin of primary haemostasis and platelet [14C]5-hydroxytryptamine release. *Br J Haematol* 1977; 36:427–436.
8. Glimelius B, Busch C, Hook M. Binding of heparin on the surface of cultured human endothelial cells. *Thromb Res* 1978; 12:773–782.
9. Mahadoo J, Heibert L, Jaques LB. Vascular sequestration of heparin. *Thromb Res* 1978; 12:79–90.
10. Ofosu FA, Sie P, Modi GJ, et al. The inhibition of thrombin-dependent positive-feedback reactions is critical to the expression of the anticoagulant effect of heparin. *Biochem J* 1987; 243:579–588.
11. Ofosu FA, Hirsh J, Esmon CT, et al. Unfractionated heparin inhibits thrombin-catalysed amplification reactions of coagulation more efficiently than those catalysed by factor Xa. *Biochem J* 1989; 257:143–150.
12. Beguin S, Lindhout T, Hemker HC. The mode of action of heparin in plasma. *Thromb Haemost* 1988; 60:457–462.
13. de Swart CA, Nijmeyer B, Roelofs JM, Sixma JJ. Kinetics of intravenously administered heparin in normal humans. *Blood* 1982; 60:1251–1258.
14. Olsson P, Lagergren H, Ek S. The elimination from plasma of intravenous heparin. An experimental study on dogs and humans. *Acta Med Scand* 1963; 173:619–630.
15. Bjornsson TO, Wolfram BS, Kitchell BB. Heparin kinetics determined by three assay methods. *Clin Pharmacol Ther* 1982; 31:104.

16. Simon TL, Hyers TM, Gaston JP, Harker LA. Heparin pharmacokinetics: increased requirements in pulmonary embolism. *Br J Haematol* 1978; 39:111–120.

17. Holt JC, Niewiarowski S. Biochemistry of alpha granule proteins. *Semin Hematol* 1985; 22:151–163.

18. Lijnen HR, Hoylaerts M, Collen D. Heparin binding properties of human histidine-rich glycoprotein. Mechanism and role in the neutralization of heparin in plasma. *J Biol Chem* 1983; 258:3803–3808.

19. Preissner KT, Muller-Berghaus G. Neutralization and binding of heparin by S protein/vitronectin in the inhibition of factor Xa by antithrombin III. Involvement of an inducible heparin-binding domain of S protein/vitronectin. *J Biol Chem* 1987; 262:12247–12253.

20. Fry ET, Sobel BE. Lack of interference by heparin with thrombolysis or binding of tissue-type plasminogen activator to thrombi. *Blood* 1988; 71:1347–1352.

21. Agnelli G, Pascucci C, Cosmi B, Nenci GG. Effects of therapeutic doses of heparin on thrombolysis with tissue-type plasminogen activator in rabbits. *Blood* 1990; 76:2030–2036.

22. Landefeld CS, Cook EF, Flatley M, Weisberg M, Goldman L. Identification and preliminary validation of predictors of major bleeding in hospitalized patients starting anticoagulant therapy. *Am J Med* 1987; 82:703–713.

23. Conti S, Daschbach M, Blaisdell FW. A comparison of high-dose versus conventional-dose heparin therapy for deep vein thrombosis. *Surgery* 1982; 92:972–980.

24. Hull RD, Raskob GE, Hirsh J, et al. Continuous intravenous heparin compared with intermittent subcutaneous heparin in the initial treatment of proximal-vein thrombosis. *N Engl J Med* 1986; 315:1109–1114.

25. Wheeler AP, Jaquiss RD, Newman JH. Physician practices in the treatment of pulmonary embolism and deep venous thrombosis. *Arch Intern Med* 1988; 148:1321–1325.

26. Hull RD, Raskob GE, Rosenbloom D, et al. Optimal therapeutic level of heparin therapy in patients with venous thrombosis. *Arch Intern Med* 1992; 152:1589–1595.

27. Hirsh J, Poller L, Deykin D, Levine M, Dalen JE. Optimal therapeutic range for oral anticoagulants. *Chest* 1989; 95:5S–11S.

28. Brandjes DP, Heijboer H, Buller HR, et al. Acenocoumarol and heparin compared with acenocoumarol alone in the initial treatment of proximal-vein thrombosis. *N Engl J Med* 1992; 327:1485–1489.

29. Bratt G, Tornebohm E, Widlund L, Lockner D. Low molecular weight heparin (KABI 2165, Fragmin): pharmacokinetics after intravenous and subcutaneous administration in human volunteers. *Thromb Res* 1986; 42:613–620.

30. Bara L, Billaud E, Gramond G, Kher A, Samama M. Comparative pharmacokinetics of a low molecular weight heparin (PK 10 169) and unfractionated heparin after intravenous and subcutaneous administration. *Thromb Res* 1985; 39:631–636.

31. van der Heijden JF, Hutten BA, Buller HR, Prins MH. Vitamin K antagonists or low-molecular-weight heparin for the long term treatment of symptomatic venous thromboembolism. *Cochrane Database Syst Rev* 2002; CD002001.

32. Hull RD, Raskob GE, Pineo GF, et al. Subcutaneous low-molecular-weight heparin compared with continuous intravenous heparin in the treatment of proximal-vein thrombosis. *N Engl J Med* 1992; 326:975–982.

33. Lee AY, Levine MN, Baker RI, et al. Low-molecular-weight heparin versus a coumarin for the prevention of recurrent venous thromboembolism in patients with cancer. *N Engl J Med* 2003; 349:146–153.

34. Boneu B, Necciari J, Cariou R, et al. Pharmacokinetics and tolerance of the natural pentasaccharide (SR90107/Org31540) with high affinity to antithrombin III in man. *Thromb Haemost* 1995; 74:1468–1473.

35. Warkentin TE. Heparin-induced thrombocytopenia associated with fondaparinux. *N Engl J Med* 2007; 356:2653–2654.

36. Turpie AG, Gallus AS, Hoek JA. A synthetic pentasaccharide for the prevention of deep-vein thrombosis after total hip replacement. *N Engl J Med* 2001; 344:619–625.

37. Greinacher A, Eichler P, Lubenow N, Kwasny H, Luz M. Heparin-induced thrombocytopenia with thromboembolic complications: meta-analysis of 2 prospective trials to assess the value of parenteral treatment with lepirudin and its therapeutic aPTT range. *Blood* 2000; 96:846–851.

38. Lewis BE. Argatroban therapy in heparin-induced thrombocytopenia. In Reinacher A (ed.), *Heparin-induced thrombocytopenia*. New York: Marcel Dekker, 2004: 437–474.

39. Arpino PA, Hallisey RK. Effect of renal function on the pharmacodynamics of argatroban. *Ann Pharmacother* 2004; 38:25–29.

40. Maraganore JM, Bourdon P, Jablonski J, Ramachandran KL, Fenton JW. Design and characterization of hirulogs: a novel class of bivalent peptide inhibitors of thrombin. *Biochemisty* 1990; 29:7095–7101.

41. Bartholomew JR. Bivalirudin for the treatment of heparin-induced thrombocytopenia. In Reinacher A (ed.), *Heparin-induced thrombocytopenia*. New York: Marcel Dekker, 2004: 475–507.

42. Francis JL, Drexler A, Gwyn G. Bivalirudin, a direct thrombin inhibitor, is a safe and effective treatment for heparin-induced thrombocytopenia (abstract). *Blood* 2003; 102:164a.

43. Furie B, Furie BC. Molecular basis of vitamin K-dependent gamma-carboxylation. *Blood* 1990; 75:1753–1762.

44. Vermeer C. Gamma-carboxyglutamate-containing proteins and the vitamin K-dependent carboxylase. *Biochem J* 1990; 266:625–636.

45. O'Reilly RA, Rytand DA. "Resistance" to warfarin due to unrecognized vitamin K supplementation. *N Engl J Med* 1980; 303:160–161.

46. Wessler S, Gitel SN. Warfarin. From bedside to bench. *N Engl J Med* 1984; 311:645–652.

47. Hellemans J, Vorlat M, Verstraete M. Survival time of prothrombin and factors VII, IX and X after completely synthesis blocking doses of coumarin derivatives. *Br J Haematol* 1963; 9:506–512.

48. Zivelin A, Rao LV, Rapaport SI. Mechanism of the anticoagulant effect of warfarin as evaluated in rabbits by selective depression of individual procoagulant vitamin K-dependent clotting factors. *J Clin Invest* 1993; 92:2131–2140.

49. Chong BH, Ismail F, Cade J, et al. Heparin-induced thrombocytopenia: studies with a new low molecular weight heparinoid, Org 10172. *Blood* 1989; 73:1592–1596.

50. Chong BH, Gallus AS, Cade JF, et al. Prospective randomised open-label comparison of danaparoid with dextran 70 in the treatment of heparin-induced thrombocytopaenia with thrombosis: a clinical outcome study. *Thromb Haemost* 2001; 86:1170–1175.

6

New oral anticoagulants

Overview

After more than half a century of anticoagulation with heparin and vitamin K antagonists (VKAs), a new generation of oral anticoagulants is becoming available. Warfarin and its related oral VKAs have been the mainstay for the management and prophylaxis of thrombosis for more than 50 years. Ansell et al.[1] have characterized the use of VKAs in clinical practice as (1) having a narrow therapeutic range, (2) exhibiting considerable variability in dose response among patients due to genetic and other factors, (3) being subject to interactions with drugs and diet, (4) having laboratory control that can be difficult to standardize, and (5) requiring an understanding of pharmacokinetics, pharmacodynamics, and good patient communication for maintenance of a sustained therapeutic level (Box 6.1).

The new oral anticoagulants (NOACs) have generated enthusiasm. The four leading NOACs are dabigatran, apixaban, edoxaban, and rivaroxaban. A number of additional drugs are in earlier stages of clinical development. Although the characteristics of the new anticoagulants are attractive and their potential ease of use welcome, it is appropriate to temper one's enthusiasm since they are new, large clinical experiences are as yet unavailable, and most clinicians have little or no experience with these drugs. A limitation and ongoing concern is that a reversal agent for these drugs has not yet been developed.

On the other hand, VKAs are familiar to most every physician. Virtually all aspects of this class of drugs are well known, including mechanism of action and metabolism, a well-recognized tool (international normalized ratio [INR]) for monitoring therapeutic levels, and uniformly available and highly effective reversal agents. Vitamin K, fresh frozen plasma, prothrombin complex concentrate, and recombinant factor VIIa have all been effective in reversing the anticoagulant effect of VKAs. Warfarin compounds are associated with serious bleeding complications; however, it is unusual for patients to develop non-bleeding-related morbidities. The first oral direct thrombin inhibitor to undergo clinical evaluation was ximelagatran.[2] It had attractive pharmacodynamics characteristics such as binding to the active site of thrombin and inactivating fibrin-bound thrombin.[3] Binding was reversible and allowed relatively quick dissociation from thrombin, permitting a small amount of thrombin to remain available for adequate hemostasis.[4] The recent experience with ximelagatran, the initial oral direct thrombin inhibitor, demonstrated effectiveness in the management of deep venous thrombosis (DVT), but a larger than anticipated number of patients developed critical increases in liver enzymes indicating hepatotoxicity,[5] which resulted in withdrawal of the drug from the market in 2006 by Astra Zeneca.[6] As a result, regulatory agencies are carefully scrutinizing data, and pharmaceutical companies and clinicians are temporizing their enthusiasm for these new agents until greater experience is obtained.

Two new direct oral anticoagulants (dabigatran and rivaroxaban) have been approved by the U.S. Food and Drug Administration (FDA) for the management of patients with nonvalvular atrial fibrillation, and two are in the late stages of clinical trials (apixaban and edoxaban). Rivaroxaban has recently been approved by the FDA for the management of patients with acute venous thromboembolism (VTE). A number of other agents are in earlier stages of development. The NOACs have a number of advantages compared to VKAs (Box 6.2).

These four drugs are summarized in Table 6.1.[7,8] These are all small molecules and readily absorbed from the gastrointestinal tract when ingested orally. Warfarin requires 4–5 days of therapy to produce a therapeutic anticoagulant effect since it functions by reducing the production of the coagulation proenzymes. However, the new agents directly inhibit factor Xa or thrombin and are rapidly active.

Dabigatran etexilate is a prodrug. Following ingestion, it is converted to dabigatran by esterases in the blood and liver.[9] The three other drugs are active in their ingested form. The metabolism of the new oral anticoagulants involves cytochrome p450 3A4, p-glycoprotein, or both. As such, patients taking concomitant agents that induce p-glycoprotein (such as rifampin) may alter the drug's activity.

Clinical trial development

The protocols used by the NOACs during their clinical trials were generally similar. Studies were designed to assess fixed doses of drug and did not include dose titration. All studies comparing the oral anticoagulants with an existing anticoagulant (enoxaparin or warfarin) were powered for noninferiority. Only studies comparing a NOAC versus a placebo were powered for superiority.

Initial studies evaluated VTE prophylaxis in orthopedic surgical patients followed by treatment and secondary prevention for patients with DVT and pulmonary embolism (PE). Since this book is focused on venous thrombosis, the important pivotal trials of these new agents that addressed thromboembolic events in patients with nonvalvular atrial fibrillation will not be addressed.

VTE prophylaxis in orthopedic patients

Venous thromboembolic complications following major orthopedic surgery are a significant postoperative concern, and low-molecular-weight heparin (LMWH) is the preferred form of routine prophylaxis.[10] The VTE risk is not limited to the perioperative procedure but persists for at least 4 weeks following hospital discharge.[11] An oral agent that is comparable in efficacy and safety to enoxaparin would be well received by patients and physicians because of greater patient comfort and anticipated improved compliance, since injections would no longer be necessary.

Dabigatran

Dabigatran has been widely studied in orthopedic surgical patients. The RE-NOVATE trial[12] studied patients undergoing total hip replacement.

Table 6.1 NOACs: Comparative pharmacology

Characteristic	Agent			
	Dabigatran	**Apixaban**	**Edoxaban**	**Rivaroxaban**
Target	Thrombin	Factor Xa	Factor Xa	Factor Xa
Prodrug	Yes	No	No	No
Bioavailability	6%	50%	100%	80%
Dosing	Fixed b.i.d.	Fixed b.i.d	Fixed q.d.	Initial b.i.d.
Formulation	Capsule with coated beads (should not be opened)	File-coated tablet (should not be crushed)	Film-coated tablet	Film-coated tablet (should not be crushed)
Tmax	1.25–6 hours	3–4 hours	1–4 hours	2–4 hours
Half-life	12–17 hours	12 hours	6–12 hours	7–11 hours
Renal clearance	80%	27%	62%	35%
Protein binding	35%	87%	40–59%	92–95%
Routine coagulation monitoring	No	No	No	No
PK-drug interactions	Quinidine, amiodarone, potent Pgp inhibitors	Potent CYP3A4 and Pgp inhibitors	Potent Pgp inhibitors	Potent CYP3A4 and Pgp inhibitors

Sources: Data from Eriksson BI, et al., *Clin Pharmacokinet* 2009; 48:1–22; Mavrakanas T, Bounameaux H, *Pharmacol Ther* 2011; 130:46–58.

The RE-MOBILIZE[13] and RE-MODEL[14] trials studied patients undergoing total knee replacement. These studies compared prophylaxis with dabigatran with the LMWH enoxaparin. Interestingly, the control arms had different enoxaparin doses, which were dictated by the local standard of care. The RE-MODEL and RE-NOVATE trials used 40 mg daily doses of enoxaparin, most likely because they were conducted in Europe. The RE-MOBILIZE trial conducted in the United States used 30 mg of enoxaparin b.i.d. Two doses of dabigatran were evaluated in all three studies, namely, 150 and 220 mg once daily. The primary endpoint for these studies was a composite of total VTE events and all-cause mortality, and safety focused on bleeding complications.

Both doses of dabigatran were found to be noninferior to 40 mg of enoxaparin daily. There were similar rates of bleeding complications. However, in the RE-MOBILIZE trial, enoxaparin 30 mg b.i.d. proved to be superior to both doses of dabigatran. Since the 30 mg b.i.d. dose of enoxaparin gives patients 50% more enoxaparin per day than the 40 mg dose, it has been recognized to be more effective and is a more stringent

comparator to the new oral anticoagulants. In all three trials there were no significant differences in bleeding rates.

Apixaban

Apixaban has been evaluated in orthopedic surgical patients in the three ADVANCE trials. The ADVANCE-1 trial compared apixaban 2.5 mg twice daily with enoxaparin 30 mg twice daily for the prevention of VTE after total knee replacement.[15] The primary efficacy endpoint was surprisingly low and similar in both groups (apixaban 9.0% vs. enoxaparin 8.8%). However, the statistical endpoint of noninferiority was not met by the smallest of margins ($p = .06$). An interesting observation was that the composite of major and clinically relevant nonmajor bleeding was significantly lower with apixaban than with enoxaparin (2.9% vs. 4.3%; $p = .03$). In the subsequent ADVANCE-2 trial[16] evaluating patients undergoing total knee replacement and the ADVANCE-3 trial,[17] which evaluated patients undergoing total hip replacement, apixaban was compared with the 40 mg daily enoxaparin dose starting 12 hours preoperatively. The primary outcome measure was the composite of symptomatic and asymptomatic DVT, nonfatal PE, and all-cause mortality. In ADVANCE-2, apixaban was significantly better than enoxaparin in reducing the primary endpoint (15% vs. 24%; RR 0.62; $p < .0001$). Major and clinically relevant nonmajor bleeding occurred in 4% of apixaban-treated patients and 5% of patients receiving enoxaparin (NS). In the ADVANCE-3 trial, which evaluated patients undergoing total hip replacement, apixaban once again demonstrated superiority versus 40 mg daily of enoxaparin (1.4% vs. 3.9%; RR 0.36; $p < .001$). The composite outcome of major and clinically relevant nonmajor bleeding was not different between the two groups.

Edoxaban

Edoxaban has been studied for VTE prophylaxis in orthopedic patients in Japan and Taiwan. Dose-ranging studies were performed in Japan to establish appropriate doses for patients undergoing total hip[18] and total knee[19] replacement. Moving into phase 3 trials, a unique dose of enoxaparin given 20 mg subcutaneously b.i.d. was compared with edoxaban 30 mg daily.

A small study that evaluated 92 patients undergoing hip fracture surgery failed to demonstrate any difference between the two treatment groups either in efficacy (edoxaban 7% vs. enoxaparin 4%) or safety.[20] There was no difference in bleeding complications.

In a larger study ($N = 610$) of patients undergoing total hip replacement, edoxaban 30 mg daily versus enoxaparin 20 mg b.i.d. was compared.[21] Edoxaban treatment resulted in a significant reduction in total venous thromboembolic events (2.4%) compared with patients receiving enoxaparin (6.9%; $p < .001$). There was no difference in bleeding complications between the two groups.

In the final edoxaban orthopedic study comparing 716 patients undergoing total knee replacement, the same doses of edoxaban and enoxaparin were used (30 mg daily and 20 mg b.i.d., respectively).[22] Venous thromboembolic events were significantly fewer in edoxaban-treated patients (7.4%) versus patients receiving enoxaparin (13.9%; $p = .01$). As in the other edoxaban trials, there was no difference in bleeding complications.

Rivaroxaban

Rivaroxaban has been evaluated for VTE prophylaxis in four trials of patients undergoing orthopedic surgery. RECORD-1[23] and RECORD-2[24] evaluated patients undergoing total hip replacement, and RECORD-3[25] and RECORD-4[26] evaluated patients undergoing total knee replacement. In three of the four RECORD trials (1–3), rivaroxaban 10 mg daily was compared with 40 mg of enoxaparin daily, and in RECORD-4 the comparator dose of enoxaparin was 30 mg twice daily.

A pooled analysis of the four studies evaluated the primary endpoint of symptomatic VTE plus all-cause mortality.[27] Safety was defined as bleeding complications. The primary efficacy endpoint occurred in 0.5% of patients on rivaroxaban versus 1% of patients taking enoxaparin (HR 0.48; $p = .001$). There was no significant difference between major and nonmajor clinically relevant bleeding.

Specific evaluation of the RECORD-4 study appears warranted, since the most effective dose of enoxaparin (30 mg q. 12 hours) was used. A total 3148 patients undergoing knee arthroplasty were randomized to oral rivaroxaban 10 mg daily versus enoxaparin 30 mg q. 12 hours.[26] The primary efficacy outcome was the composite of any DVT (symptomatic or asymptomatic), nonfatal PE, or all-cause mortality up to day 17 after surgery. The primary efficacy endpoint was reached in 6.9% of rivaroxaban-treated patients versus 10.1% of those treated with enoxaparin ($p = .0118$). Although there were numerically more bleeding events with rivaroxaban, the difference compared with enoxaparin was not significant.

VTE prophylaxis in medically ill patients

Venous thromboembolic complications commonly complicate the hospital course of acutely ill medical patients. The benefits of providing pharmacologic prophylaxis during hospitalization have been previously described in randomized trials.[28,29] Current guidelines suggest that high-risk medical patients be protected with pharmacologic thromboprophylaxis if not at high risk for bleeding.[30]

Two prospective randomized trials have been performed using the new oral anticoagulants in high-risk medically ill patients.

The MAGELLAN trial[31] evaluated rivaroxaban for thrombosis prophylaxis in medically ill patients. This was a two-part study. In part 1, 10 mg of rivaroxaban daily was compared with 40 mg of enoxaparin daily in high-risk medical patients. At day 10, rivaroxaban met its primary clinical efficacy objective of demonstrating noninferiority to enoxaparin in short-term use; both groups had a thrombosis rate of 2.7%. However, the rate of bleeding was higher with rivaroxaban than enoxaparin (2.8% vs. 1.2%).

Part 2 of the study extended rivaroxaban to 35 days versus placebo. The results demonstrated that the combined rates of major and clinically relevant nonmajor bleeding, the primary safety measure in this study, while low overall, were significantly higher in those treated with rivaroxaban than in those treated with enoxaparin followed by placebo.

The ADOPT trial investigators[32] studied apixaban versus enoxaparin for thromboprophylaxis in medically ill patients. This was a double-blind, double-dummy, placebo-controlled trial that randomly assigned acutely ill medical patients to receive apixaban 2.5 mg twice daily × 30 days or enoxaparin 40 mg once daily for 6–14 days. The primary efficacy outcome was the 30-day composite of death related to VTE, PE, symptomatic DVT, or asymptomatic proximal DVT (detected by compression ultrasonography) on day 30. The primary safety outcome was bleeding.

A total 6528 subjects were randomized. The primary efficacy outcome was achieved in 2.71% of apixaban-treated patients and 3.06% in the enoxaparin group. Relative risk for apixaban was 0.87 (p = .44 for superiority). By day 30, major bleeding occurred in 0.47% of the apixaban group and 0.19% of the enoxaparin group. On the basis of these observations, the investigators concluded that an extended course of thromboprophylaxis with apixaban was not superior to a shorter course of enoxaparin in medically ill patients. Apixaban was associated with more bleeding events than was enoxaparin.

To date, in acutely ill medical patients, extended (postdischarge) prophylaxis with the NOACs has not been shown to be more effective than shorter-term enoxaparin.

Treatment of acute VTE

Patients with acute VTE are most commonly treated with heparin followed by VKAs. VKAs require frequent monitoring using the INR, and as previously discussed, there are multiple interactions with food and other drugs. The NOACs do not require monitoring, have minimal food and drug interactions, and therefore are thought to be attractive alternatives to VKAs in the management of patients with acute VTE. An overview of the clinical trials for the early treatment and extended prophylaxis of acute VTE is provided in Tables 6.2[33–39] and 6.3.[40–42]

Dabigatran

The RE-COVER study group evaluated dabigatran versus warfarin in the treatment of acute VTE.[33] These investigators randomized 2564 patients to receive oral dabigatran 150 mg twice daily or warfarin that was dose-adjusted to achieve an INR of 2.0–3.0. All patients received parenteral anticoagulation for a median of 9 days. The primary outcomes were the 6-month incidence of recurrent, symptomatic, objectively confirmed VTE and death. Safety endpoints included bleeding events, acute coronary syndromes, other adverse events, and results of liver function tests.

Recurrent VTE occurred in 2.4% of dabigatran patients versus 2.1% of those receiving warfarin. This achieved a p value of 0.001 for the prespecified noninferiority margin. There was no difference in major bleeding complications. There was a significant reduction in all-cause bleeding in patients randomized to dabigatran.

Significantly more patients randomized to dabigatran discontinued their study drug, presumably due to dyspepsia, which was more frequent in this cohort of patients than those randomized to warfarin. There were no differences in liver enzyme elevation.

The results of the RE-COVER study demonstrated that a fixed dose of dabigatran is as effective as warfarin for the management of patients with acute VTE and has a safety profile similar to that of warfarin but does not require laboratory monitoring.

The RE-COVER II[34] trial was a similarly designed and performed trial to RE-COVER, although the

Table 6.2 NOACs: Summary of trials for the treatment of acute VTE

Trial	Design time	Drug	Comparator	Patients	Recurrent VTE NOAC vs. comparator (%)	Major bleeding p value
RE-COVER[33]	Double-blind 6 months	LMWH or UFH Dabigatran 150 mg b.i.d.	LMWH or UFH/warfarin	2539	2.4 vs. 2.1 p < .001 (noninferior)	1.6 vs. 1.9 NS
RE-COVER II[34]	Double-blind 6 months	LMWH or UFH Dabigatran 150 mg b.i.d.	LMWH or UFH/warfarin	2568	2.4 vs. 2.2 p < .001 (noninferior)	1.2 vs. 1.7 NS
EINSTEIN DVT[35]	Open label 3, 6, or 12 months	Rivaroxaban 15 mg b.i.d. × 21 days, then 20 mg o.d.	Enoxaparin/ warfarin	3449	2.1 vs. 2.0 p < .001 (noninferior)	0.8 vs. 1.2 p = .21
EINSTEIN PE[36]	Open label 3, 6, or 12 months	Rivaroxaban 15 mg b.i.d. × 21 days, then 20 mg o.d.	Enoxaparin/ warfarin	4833	2.1 vs. 1.8 p < .0028 (noninferior)	1.1 vs. 2.2 p = .0032
AMPLIFY[37]	Double-blind 6 months	Apixaban 10 mg b.i.d. × 7 days, then 5 mg b.i.d.	Enoxaparin/ warfarin	4616	2.3 vs. 2.7 p < .001 (noninferior)	0.6 vs 1.8 p < .001
HOKUSAI[38]	Double-blind <12 months	LMWH or UFH edoxaban 60 mg o.d.	LMWH or UFH/warfarin	7500	Ongoing	Ongoing

Sources: Data from Becattini C, et al., *Thromb Res* 2012; 129:392–400. Agnelli G, et al., *N Engl J Med* 07.01.13 epub. Available at http://www.nejm.org/doi/full/10.1056/NEJMoa1302507. Accessed 07/11/13.

population of patients was somewhat different in that more Asians took part. Results were also similar; dabigatran 150 mg b.i.d. was found to be noninferior to warfarin for the management of acute VTE. Recurrent VTE occurred in 2.4% of patients randomized to dabigatran and 2.2% randomized to warfarin ($p < .0001$ for noninferiority). Major bleeding and any bleeding were not different between groups. Rates of recurrent VTE and any bleeding were similar in Asian and non-Asian patients.

The RE-SONATE investigators[40] performed a double-blind placebo-controlled trial of 6 months of extended therapy with dabigatran 150 mg p.o. b.i.d. versus placebo in 1343 patients following 6–18 months of therapeutic anticoagulation for acute VTE. The primary outcome of symptomatic recurrent VTE and VTE-related death was significantly reduced in the treatment group (0.4%) versus those receiving placebo (5.6%; $p < .0001$).

However, there was an increased risk of major bleeding and clinically relevant nonmajor bleeding with dabigatran (1.8% vs. 5.3%; $p < .001$).

In another extended treatment trial, the REMEDY investigators[40] evaluated the same dose of dabigatran to warfarin for up to 36 months. The primary outcome was a composite of symptomatic recurrent VTE and VTE-related death. There was no difference in outcome between groups (1.85 vs. 1.3%; $p = .03$ for noninferiority). However, there was more major and clinically relevant nonmajor bleeding with warfarin (10.2% vs. 5.6%; $p = .001$).

Apixaban

The AMPLIFY investigators[37] conducted a double-blind, noninferiority study in 5395 patients with acute VTE evaluating apixaban 10 mg b.i.d. × 7

Table 6.3 NOACs: Summary of extended treatment trials

Trial	Design time	Drug	Comparator	Patients	Recurrent VTE NOAC vs. comparator (%)	Major bleeding p value
RE-MEDY[40]	Double-blind 36 months	Dabigatran 150 mg b.i.d.	Warfarin; INR 2.0–3.0	2850 pretreatment 3–12 months	1.8 vs. 1.3 p = .03 (noninferior)	0.8 vs. 1.8 p = .058
RE-SONATE[40]	Double-blind 6 months	Dabigatran 150 mg b.i.d.	Placebo	1343 pretreatment 6–18 months	0.4 vs. 5.6 p < .001	0.3 vs. 0 p = .986
EINSTEIN-EXTENSION[41]	Double-blind 6–12 months	Rivaroxaban 20 mg o.d.	Placebo	1196 pretreatment <12 months	1.3 vs. 7.1 p = .001	0.7 vs. 0 p = .11
AMPLIFY-EXTENSION[42]	Double-blind 12 months	Apixaban 2.5 mg/5.0 mg daily	Placebo	2486 randomized	(2.5 mg) 1.7 vs. 7.0 (5.0 mg) 1.7 vs. .7.0 p < .001 for both	(2.5 mg) 0.2 vs. 0.5 (5.0 mg) 0.1 vs. 0.5 p = NS for both

Sources: Data from Becattini C, et al., *Thromb Res* 2012; 129:392–400; Agnelli G, et al. *N Engl J Med* 2013; 368:699–708.

days followed by 5 mg b.i.d. for 6 months versus initial enoxaparin followed by warfarin adjusted to an INR of 2.0–3.0. The primary efficacy outcome measures were recurrent VTE or death, and the primary safety outcomes were major and clinically relevant nonmajor bleeding. The primary efficacy outcome occurred in 2.3% of the apixaban group versus 2.7% in the conventional therapy group (relative risk 0.84). Apixaban was noninferior to conventional therapy (p = .001). Major bleeding occurred in 0.6% receiving apixaban and 1.8% receiving conventional treatment (relative risk 0.31; p < .001 for superiority). The composite outcome of major and clinically relevant nonmajor bleeding occurred in 4.3% of the apixaban group and 9.7% of the conventional treatment group (relative risk 0.44; p <.001).

The AMPLIFY-EXTENSION trial[42] compared two doses of apixaban (2.5 or 5 mg b.i.d.) with placebo for the prevention of recurrent VTE over a 12-month period in patients who had completed an initial course of treatment for VTE and if there was clinical equipoise about the continuation or cessation of anticoagulant therapy. Additional aims of the study were to determine whether the 2.5 mg dose of apixaban was effective and associated with less bleeding than the 5 mg dose, and to examine the effect of extended treatment on arterial thrombotic outcomes.

The primary efficacy outcome was the composite of symptomatic recurrent VTE or death from any cause. An additional efficacy outcome was the composite of symptomatic recurrent VTE, death related to VTE, myocardial infarction, stroke, or death related to cardiovascular disease. The primary safety outcome was major bleeding. The secondary safety outcome was the composite of major or clinically relevant nonmajor bleeding.

A total 2486 patients were randomized. Symptomatic recurrent VTE or death from VTE occurred in 8.8% receiving placebo compared with 1.7% who were receiving 2.5 mg of apixaban and 1.7% who were receiving 5 mg of apixaban (p < .001). The rates of major bleeding were 0.5% in the placebo group, 0.2% in the 2.5 mg apixaban group, and 0.1% in the 5 mg apixaban group (p = NS). The remaining data are summarized in Table 6.4.[42]

The number of patients needed to be treated to prevent one episode of recurrent VTE during the 1-year active study period was 14, whereas the number needed for treatment to cause one episode of major or clinically relevant nonmajor bleeding was 200.

The conclusions of this study were that extended anticoagulation with apixaban at either the 2.5 mg or 5 mg dose reduced the risk of recurrent VTE without increasing the rate of major bleeding.

Table 6.4 Clinical outcomes in the apixaban extended study: intention-to-treat analysis

	Treatment		
Outcome	Placebo (N = 829)	Apixaban 2.5 mg (N = 840)	Apixaban 5.0 mg (N = 813)
Primary endpoint	11.6%	3.8%	4.2%
Symptomatic recurrent VTE or VTE-related death	8.8%	1.7%	1.7%
Symptomatic VTE, VTE death, myocardial infarction (MI), stroke, cardiovascular (CV) death	10%	2.1%	2.3%
MI, stroke, CV death	1.3%	0.5%	0.6%
Major bleeding	0.5%	0.2%	0.1%
Clinically relevant nonmajor bleeding	2.3%	3.0%	4.2%
Major and clinically relevant nonmajor bleeding	2.7%	3.2%	4.3%
VTE, VTE death, MI, stroke, CV death, or major bleeding	10.4%	2.4%	2.5%

Source: Data from Agnelli G, et al., *N Engl J Med* 2013; 368:699–708.

The 2.5 mg dose had an overall bleeding profile similar to that of placebo.

Edoxaban

The HOUKUSAI investigators[38] are performing a double-blind study comparing LMWH or unfractionated heparin (UFH) followed by edoxaban 60 mg daily to LMWH or UFH followed by warfarin for patients with acute VTE. Over 7500 patients have been randomized. The primary endpoint is recurrent VTE with the safety endpoint being bleeding complications. This study is currently ongoing.

Rivaroxaban

The EINSTEIN investigators[35] evaluated rivaroxaban versus standard anticoagulation in a two-phased study in patients with acute symptomatic VTE. Phase 1 randomized 3449 patients with acute DVT to either rivaroxaban 50 mg b.i.d. × 3 weeks followed by 20 mg daily versus enoxaparin × 5 days followed by warfarin. This study had a noninferiority design with the primary endpoint being recurrent VTE and the safety endpoint being bleeding. Results demonstrated that recurrence occurred in 2.1% of the rivaroxaban group versus 3% of the enoxaparin/VKA-treated patients ($p < .001$ for noninferiority; $p = .08$ for superiority). There was no difference in bleeding complications.

Phase 2 of the study was a continued treatment study randomizing 1196 patients with acute DVT who had completed a 6- to 12-month course of standard anticoagulation. They were randomized in a double-blind fashion to rivaroxaban 20 mg daily versus placebo. This study was designed as a superiority trial, with the primary endpoint being recurrent VTE with a safety endpoint of bleeding.

The results of the phase 2 study demonstrated that rivaroxaban was superior to placebo. Recurrent VTE occurred in 7.1% of the placebo group versus 1.3% of the rivaroxaban group ($p < .001$ for superiority). There was no significant difference in bleeding between the two treatment groups.

The authors concluded that in the initial phase of managing acute VTE, rivaroxaban was equivalent to heparin followed by VKAs but did not require laboratory monitoring. However, in the continued treatment study, rivaroxaban significantly reduced recurrent VTE without increasing the risk of bleeding.

The Einstein PE trial[36] compared rivaroxaban 15 mg b.i.d. × 21 days followed by 20 mg once daily for the intended treatment period of 3, 6, or 12 months versus standard anticoagulation (LMWH followed by VKAs) in patients with acute symptomatic PE with or without symptomatic DVT. The primary efficacy endpoint was prevention of symptomatic VTE. Rivaroxaban was noninferior to standard therapy (2.1% vs. 1.8%; $p = .003$ for noninferiority). Major or clinically relevant nonmajor bleeding occurred in 10.3% of patients in the rivaroxaban group and 11.4% of patients in the standard therapy group ($p = .23$). However, major bleeding was observed less frequently in the rivaroxaban group compared with standard therapy (1.1% vs. 2.2%; $p = .003$). These data lend further evidence that many patients with symptomatic PE can be effectively and safely managed as outpatients.

Rivaroxaban is the first NOAC to be approved in the United States for the treatment of acute VTE. As of this writing, no other agent has received approval.

Reversal of the anticoagulant effect of NOACs

The NOACs have a relatively short half-life. Most prospective studies have demonstrated no increased risk of major bleeding compared to VKAs. Actually, less major bleeding and clinically relevant nonmajor bleeding have been observed with the NOACs. However, physicians continue to be concerned about the lack of a reversal agent in the rare patient who may require immediate reversal of their anticoagulant effect. An overview of reversal of antiocoagulants is summarized in Table 6.5.[43] Hypothetically, prothrombin complex concentrate (PCC) should overcome the anticoagulant effect induced by both thrombin inhibitors and factor Xa inhibitors since it contains the coagulation factors II, VII, IX, and X in high concentration and generally increases thrombin generation.[44]

Table 6.5 Bleeding and time to reversal of anticoagulation by agent

Agent	Time until restoration	Active reversal	Comment
VKA	Warfarin 60–80 hours	VKA IV in 12–16 hours	VKA/PCC/FFP dose depends on INR and weight
	Acenocumarol 18–24 hours	VKA p.o. in 24 hours	
		PCC: immediate	
		Fresh frozen plasma: immediate	
Pentasaccharide	Fondaparinux 24–30 hours	Recombinant FVIIa immediate	Monitored with laboratory endpoints
FXa inhibitors	Depends on agent; usually approximately 12 hours	Prothrombin complex concentrate	Monitored with laboratory endpoints
Direct thrombin inhibitors	Depends on agent; usually approximately 12 hours	Nine at present (PCC not effective)	

Source: Data from Levi M, et al., *J Thromb Haemost* 2011; 9:1705–1712.

Eerenberg et al.[45] studied the use of PCC in subjects receiving rivaroxaban and dabigatran on reversal of the anticoagulation effect of these drugs in a randomized, placebo-controlled, crossover study in healthy subjects. This well-designed study investigated coagulation parameters of 12 healthy male volunteers who received rivaroxaban 20 mg twice daily (N = 6) or dabigatran 150 mg twice daily (N = 6) for 2.5 days followed by either a single bolus of 50 U/kg PCC (Cofact) or a similar volume of saline. After a washout period the procedure was repeated with the subject crossing over to the other anticoagulant treatment. Both rivaroxaban and dabigatran produced a therapeutic anticoagulant effect. Rivaroxaban was immediately and completely reversed by PCC, whereas in the dabigatran-treated patients, administration of PCC did not restore the anticoagulation tests to normal. While coagulation assays are surrogate markers for a bleeding tendency and these subjects did not experience clinical bleeding, it is anticipated that there would be clinical utility for the use of PCC in patients receiving rivaroxaban and probably other direct Xa inhibitors. It is unclear why PCC did not neutralize the anticoagulant effect of the direct thrombin inhibitor since it contains a high concentration of factor II.

An accompanying commentary to the article by Eerenberg et al. was written by Elizabeth M. Battinelli.[46] She offers additional insight into the mechanism of anticoagulant reversal and further details of the randomized trials.

In addition to PCC, recombinant factor VIIa may be potentially helpful. This agent achieves hemostasis by activating thrombin on the surface of platelets. While anecdotal benefits have been observed in some patients with life-threatening bleeding, the use of recombinant activated factor VII has had inconsistent results in patients receiving other direct thrombin inhibitors.[47]

A final option available for reversal of the anticoagulant effect of dabigatran is dialysis. In an open-label study, six patients on hemodialysis for end-stage renal disease were given dabigatran. It was estimated that 62% of the drug could be removed by dialysis within 2 hours of administration.[48] However, drugs that are highly protein bound, such as rivaroxaban, will not be eliminated with hemodialysis.

Information is beginning to emerge indicating that there is no increased risk of bleeding in patients undergoing major surgery or those having emergency surgery who are treated with the NOACs versus warfarin. An analysis of over 7500 patients in the RE-LY trial[49] who underwent major or emergency surgery while being treated with dabigatron or warfarin demonstrated no difference in the rate of major or fatal bleeding between warfarin- and dabigatron-treated patients. Likewise, there was no difference in thromboembolic events. However, because of ease of use and short half-life, the dabigatran-treated patients were four times more likely to have their procedure completed within 48 hours of discontinuing their drug compared to warfarin-treated patients.

In an everyday clinical practice post-approval nationwide study of 13,914 propensity-matched patients taking either warfarin or dabigatran for atrial fibrillation, the investigators found no evidence of excess bleeding or myocardial infarction (MI) rates with dabigatran.[50] However, the dabigatran-treated patients had less mortality, intracranial bleeding, PE, and MI.

While very few patients will likely require immediate reversal of the anticoagulant effect of the NOACs, it appears that PCC is a viable option, at least for the direct Xa inhibitors. Investigation continues with the goal of developing specific antidotes for the NOACs.

REFERENCES

1. Ansell J, Hirsh J, Hylek E, Jacobson A, Crowther M, Palareti G. Pharmacology and management of the vitamin K antagonists: American College of Chest Physicians Evidence-Based Clinical Practice Guidelines (8th edition). *Chest* 2008; 133: 160S–198S.
2. Gustafsson D, Bylund R, Antonsson T, et al. A new oral anticoagulant: the 50-year challenge. *Nat Rev Drug Discov* 2004; 3:649–659.
3. Hauptmann J, Sturzebecher J. Synthetic inhibitors of thrombin and factor Xa: from bench to bedside. *Thromb Res* 1999; 93:203–241.
4. Gustafsson D, Elg M. The pharmacodynamics and pharmacokinetics of the oral direct thrombin inhibitor ximelagatran and its active metabolite melagatran: a mini-review. *Thromb Res* 2003; 109(Suppl 1):S9–S15.
5. Kindmark A, Jawaid A, Harbron CG, et al. Genome-wide pharmacogenetic investigation of a hepatic adverse event without clinical signs of immunopathology suggests an underlying immune pathogenesis. *Pharmacogenomics J* 2008; 8:186–195.
6. AstraZeneca. AstraZeneca decides to withdraw exanta (online media release). http://www.astrazeneca com/Media/Press-releases/Article/20060214—AstraZeneca-Decides-to-Withdraw-Exanta (accessed November 27, 2012).
7. Eriksson BI, Quinlan DJ, Weitz JI. Comparative pharmacodynamics and pharmacokinetics of oral direct thrombin and factor Xa inhibitors in development. *Clin Pharmacokinet* 2009; 48:1–22.
8. Mavrakanas T, Bounameaux H. The potential role of new oral anticoagulants in the prevention and treatment of thromboembolism. *Pharmacol Ther* 2011; 130:46–58.
9. Eriksson BI, Quinlan DJ, Eikelboom JW. Novel oral factor Xa and thrombin inhibitors in the management of thromboembolism. *Annu Rev Med* 2011; 62:41–57.
10. Falck-Ytter Y, Francis CW, Johanson NA, et al. Prevention of VTE in orthopedic surgery patients: Antithrombotic Therapy and Prevention of Thrombosis, 9th ed: American College of Chest Physicians Evidence-Based Clinical Practice Guidelines. *Chest* 2012; 141:e278S–e325S.
11. Planes A, Vochelle N, Darmon JY, Fagola M, Bellaud M, Huet Y. Risk of deep-venous thrombosis after hospital discharge in patients having undergone total hip replacement: double-blind randomised comparison of enoxaparin versus placebo. *Lancet* 1996; 348:224–228.
12. Eriksson BI, Dahl OE, Rosencher N, et al. Dabigatran etexilate versus enoxaparin for prevention of venous thromboembolism after total hip replacement: a randomised, double-blind, non-inferiority trial. *Lancet* 2007; 370:949–956.
13. Ginsberg JS, Davidson BL, Comp PC, et al. Oral thrombin inhibitor dabigatran etexilate vs North American enoxaparin regimen for prevention of venous thromboembolism after knee arthroplasty surgery. *J Arthroplasty* 2009; 24:1–9.
14. Eriksson BI, Dahl OE, Rosencher N, et al. Oral dabigatran etexilate vs. subcutaneous enoxaparin for the prevention of venous thromboembolism after total knee replacement: the RE-MODEL randomized trial. *J Thromb Haemost* 2007; 5:2178–2185.
15. Lassen MR, Raskob GE, Gallus A, Pineo G, Chen D, Portman RJ. Apixaban or enoxaparin for thromboprophylaxis after knee replacement. *N Engl J Med* 2009; 361:594–604.

16. Lassen MR, Raskob GE, Gallus A, Pineo G, Chen D, Hornick P. Apixaban versus enoxaparin for thromboprophylaxis after knee replacement (ADVANCE-2): a randomised double-blind trial. *Lancet* 2010; 375: 807–815.

17. Lassen MR, Gallus A, Raskob GE, Pineo G, Chen D, Ramirez LM. Apixaban versus enoxaparin for thromboprophylaxis after hip replacement. *N Engl J Med* 2010; 363: 2487–2498.

18. Raskob G, Cohen AT, Eriksson BI, et al. Oral direct factor Xa inhibition with edoxaban for thromboprophylaxis after elective total hip replacement. A randomised double-blind dose-response study. *Thromb Haemost* 2010; 104:642–649.

19. Fuji T, Fujita S, Tachibana S, Kawai Y. A dose-ranging study evaluating the oral factor Xa inhibitor edoxaban for the prevention of venous thromboembolism in patients undergoing total knee arthroplasty. *J Thromb Haemost* 2010; 8:2458–2468.

20. Fujita S, Fuji T, Tachibana S, Nakamura M, Kawai Y. Safety and efficacy of edoxaban in patients underoing hip fracture surgery (abstract). *Pathophysiol Haemost Thromb* 2010; 37:P366.

21. Fuji T, Fujita S, Tachibana S, et al. Efficacy and safety of edoxaban versus enoxaparin for the prevention of venous thromboembolism following total hip arthroplasty: STARS J-V trial (abstract). *Blood* 2010; 116:3320.

22. Fuji T, Wang CJ, Fujita S, Tachibana S, Kawai Y, Koretsune Y. Edoxaban versus enoxaparin for thromboprophylaxis after total knee arthroplasty: the STARS E-3 trial (abstract). *Pathophysiol Haemost Thromb* 2010; 37: OC297.

23. Eriksson BI, Borris LC, Friedman RJ, et al. Rivaroxaban versus enoxaparin for thromboprophylaxis after hip arthroplasty. *N Engl J Med* 2008; 358:2765–2775.

24. Kakkar AK, Brenner B, Dahl OE, et al. Extended duration rivaroxaban versus short-term enoxaparin for the prevention of venous thromboembolism after total hip arthroplasty: a double-blind, randomised controlled trial. *Lancet* 2008; 372:31–39.

25. Lassen MR, Ageno W, Borris LC, et al. Rivaroxaban versus enoxaparin for thromboprophylaxis after total knee arthroplasty. *N Engl J Med* 2008; 358:2776–2786.

26. Turpie AG, Lassen MR, Davidson BL, et al. Rivaroxaban versus enoxaparin for thromboprophylaxis after total knee arthroplasty (RECORD4): a randomised trial. *Lancet* 2009; 373:1673–1680.

27. Turpie AG, Lassen MR, Eriksson BI, et al. Rivaroxaban for the prevention of venous thromboembolism after hip or knee arthroplasty. Pooled analysis of four studies. *Thromb Haemost* 2011; 105:444–453.

28. Samama MM, Cohen AT, Darmon JY, et al. A comparison of enoxaparin with placebo for the prevention of venous thromboembolism in acutely ill medical patients. Prophylaxis in Medical Patients with Enoxaparin Study Group. *N Engl J Med* 1999; 341:793–800.

29. Leizorovicz A, Cohen AT, Turpie AG, Olsson CG, Vaitkus PT, Goldhaber SZ. Randomized, placebo-controlled trial of dalteparin for the prevention of venous thromboembolism in acutely ill medical patients. *Circulation* 2004; 110:874–879.

30. Kahn SR, Lim W, Dunn AS, et al. Prevention of VTE in nonsurgical patients: Antithrombotic Therapy and Prevention of Thrombosis, 9th ed: American College of Chest Physicians Evidence-Based Clinical Practice Guidelines. *Chest* 2012; 141:e195S–e226S.

31. Rivaroxaban compares favorably with enoxaparin in preventing venous thromboembolism in acutely ill patients without showing a net clinical benefit. American College of Cardiology, April 5, 2011. http://www.cardiosource.org/News-Media/Media-Center/News-Releases/2011/04/MAGEL-LAN.aspx.

32. Goldhaber SZ, Leizorovicz A, Kakkar AK, et al. Apixaban versus enoxaparin for thromboprophylaxis in medically ill patients. *N Engl J Med* 2011; 365:2167–2177.

33. Schulman S, Kearon C, Kakkar AK, et al. Dabigatran versus warfarin in the treatment of acute venous thromboembolism. *N Engl J Med* 2009; 361:2342–2352.

34. Schulman S, Kakkar AK, Schellong S. A randomized trial of dabigatran versus warfarin in the treatment of acute venous thromboembolism (RE-COVER II). In *Proceedings of American Society of Hematology Conference*, 2011: abstract 205.

35. Bauersachs R, Berkowitz SD, Brenner B, et al. Oral rivaroxaban for symptomatic venous thromboembolism. *N Engl J Med* 2010; 363:2499–2510.

36. Buller HR, Prins MH, Lensin AW, et al. Oral rivaroxaban for the treatment of symptomatic pulmonary embolism. *N Engl J Med* 2012; 366:1287–1297.

37. Schulman S, Eriksson H, Goldhaber SZ. Dabigatran or warfarin for extended maintenance therapy of venous thromboembolism (abstract). *J Thromb Haemost* 2011; 9:731–732.

38. Comparative investigation of low molecular weight (LMW) heparin/edoxaban tosylate (DU176b) versus (LMW) heparin/warfarin in the treatment of symptomatic deep-vein blood clots and/or lung blood clots. The Edoxaban Hokusai-VTE Study. http://clinicaltrials gov/show/NCT00986154 (accessed November 28, 2012).

39. Becattini C, Vedovati MC, Agnelli G. Old and new oral anticoagulants for venous thromboembolism and atrial fibrillation: a review of the literature. *Thromb Res* 2012; 129:392–400.

40. Schulman S, Kearon C, Kakkar AK, et al. Extended use of dabigatran, warfarin, or placebo in venous thromboembolism. *N Engl J Med* 2013;368:709-18.

41. Romualdi E, Donadini MP, Ageno W. Oral rivaroxaban after symptomatic venous thromboembolism: the continued treatment study (EINSTEIN-extension study). *Expert Rev Cardiovasc Ther* 2011; 9:841–844.

42. Efficacy and safety study of apixaban for the treatment of deep vein thrombosis or pulmonary embolism. http://clinicaltrials gov/ct2/show/NCT00643201 (accessed November 27, 2012).

43. Levi M, Eerenberg E, Kamphuisen PW. Bleeding risk and reversal strategies for old and new anticoagulants and antiplatelet agents. *J Thromb Haemost* 2011; 9:1705–1712.

44. Pezborn E, Trabandt A, Selbach K, Tinel H. Prothrombin complex concentrate reverses the effects of high-dose rivaroxaban in rats (abstract). *Pathophysiol Haemost Thromb* 2010; 37:A10-OC251.

45. Eerenberg ES, Kamphuisen PW, Sijpkens MK, Meijers JC, Buller HR, Levi M. Reversal of rivaroxaban and dabigatran by prothrombin complex concentrate: a randomized, placebo-controlled, crossover study in healthy subjects. *Circulation* 2011; 124:1573–1579.

46. Battinelli EM. Reversal of new oral anticoagulants. *Circulation* 2011; 124:1508–1510.

47. van RJ, Stangier J, Haertter S, et al. Dabigatran etexilate—a novel, reversible, oral direct thrombin inhibitor: interpretation of coagulation assays and reversal of anticoagulant activity. *Thromb Haemost* 2010; 103:1116–1127.

48. Stangier J, Rathgen K, Stahle H, Mazur D. Influence of renal impairment on the pharmacokinetics and pharmacodynamics of oral dabigatran etexilate: an open-label, parallel-group, single-centre study. *Clin Pharmacokinet* 2010; 49:259–268.

49. Healey JS, Eikelboom J, Douketis J, et al. Periprocedural bleeding and thrombembolic events with dabigatran compared with warfarin. *Circulation* 2012; 126:343–348.

50. Larsen TB, Rasmussen LH, Skjoth F, et al. Efficacy and safety of dabigatran etexilate and warfarin in "real-world" patients with atrial fibrillation. *J Am Coll Cardiol* 2013; 61:2264–2273.

7

Management of acute DVT: Anticoagulation

Overview

The majority of patients with acute deep vein thrombosis (DVT) are treated with anticoagulation alone. The objectives of early anticoagulation are to stop thrombus propagation, minimize the risk of embolization, and minimize the risk of early and late recurrent DVT. The objective of long-term anticoagulation is to reduce recurrence.

Barritt and Jordan[1] performed the first and most fundamental study defining the importance of therapeutic anticoagulation for patients with venous thromboembolism (VTE). It is difficult to find another study that has had as durable an impact on the management of VTE (or any other disease process) and which has contributed to saving more lives than their paper published in *Lancet* in 1960. The first phase of their classic trial consisted of 35 patients who presented with pulmonary embolism (PE). Although PE was the initial presentation, this study serves as an important guideline illustrating the benefit of therapeutic anticoagulation for all patients with VTE. The study was designed to examine the potential benefit of anticoagulation in the management of patients with symptomatic PE.

Of the 35 patients, 16 were randomized to intravenous unfractionated heparin (UFH) followed by 14 days of warfarin anticoagulation. Nineteen patients received placebo. In this phase I trial, 53% of patients in the placebo group developed recurrent VTE versus 0% in the anticoagulation group ($p = .0005$). Twenty-six percent in the placebo group suffered a fatal PE following randomization,

compared to none receiving anticoagulation ($p = .03$). There was no difference in bleeding complications between the two groups. The ethics committee overseeing this study stopped the placebo phase of the trial and recommended that the investigators continue with phase II.

Phase II of the study expanded the anticoagulation group to 54 patients as a prospective treatment cohort and eliminated the placebo group. In the expanded anticoagulation cohort, one patient (2%) developed recurrent PE versus the 53% percent previously observed in the placebo group ($p < .0001$). There was no fatal PE in the anticoagulation group compared to the previously observed 26% in the placebo group ($p = .0007$). All-cause mortality was 26% in the placebo group versus 4% in the anticoagulation group ($p = .011$) (Table 7.1). This classic trial will never be repeated because of the adverse outcomes observed in the placebo group and because subsequent nonrandomized observational studies of untreated patients with PE yielded similar outcomes. The benefit of early anticoagulation was established.

The study by Barritt and Jordan demonstrated that initial anticoagulation with heparin followed by oral anticoagulation with a vitamin K antagonist (VKA) resulted in a marked reduction in fatal and nonfatal recurrent PE. They suggested an algorithm for dose adjustment of VKA based upon the prothrombin time. Although this study specifically addressed the management of acute PE, it is included here because it demonstrated the effectiveness of anticoagulation in the management of

Table 7.1 Anticoagulation for PE: Results of a randomized phase I trial and prospective nonrandomized phase II study

	Placebo (*N* = 19)	Anticoagulation (*N* = 54)	*p* Value
Recurrent PE	53%	2%	<.0001
Fatal PE	26%	0%	.0007
Mortality (all)	26%	4%	.011

Source: Data from Barritt DW, Jordan SC, *Lancet* 1960; 1:1309–1312.

acute symptomatic venous thromboembolic events and because of the landmark nature of the study.

Initial anticoagulation

The importance of early *therapeutic* anticoagulation has been emphasized in a number of trials.[2–4] Brandjes et al.[2] randomized patients to initial anticoagulation with heparin followed by VKAs versus initiating anticoagulation with VKA alone. They demonstrated that recurrent VTE occurred three times more frequently when patients did not receive initial therapeutic anticoagulation. This is likely due to the nontherapeutic effect of warfarin compounds early in the course of treatment.

The importance of *sustained therapeutic anticoagulation* was underscored by Hull et al.[3] when they observed a 24.5% recurrent VTE rate in patients whose heparin effect fell below therapeutic levels within the first 24 hours of therapy compared to a 1.6% recurrence rate in patients with sustained therapeutic anticoagulation (*p* < .001). This 15-fold increased risk of recurrence serves to emphasize the importance of a sustained therapeutic anticoagulant effect once treatment is initiated. Unfortunately, the link between recurrent VTE and subtherapeutic early anticoagulation is not recognized by most physicians because the recurrence does not occur immediately but rather months later.

The issue of subcutaneous low-molecular-weight heparin (LMWH) versus intravenous UFH has been addressed by numerous randomized trials and has been reviewed by the Cochrane collaborators. Van Dongen et al.[5] and Othieno et al.[6] found that LMWH was more effective than UFH for the initial treatment of DVT. They found that LMWH reduced major hemorrhage during initial treatment, reduced overall mortality, and was amenable to home therapy.

The current guidelines from the American College of Chest Physicians (ACCP)[7] addressing initial anticoagulation for acute DVT are briefly summarized in Table 7.2. The guidelines indicate that LMWH is preferred over UFH in the early treatment of acute DVT, and further state that at least 5 days of heparin overlap with a VKA is required. This duration of overlap is important to ensure therapeutic anticoagulation. The international normalized ratio (INR) can be prolonged early in the course of treatment with VKAs as a result of depletion of labile clotting factors such as factor VII. However, it is not until the levels of factors X and II are depressed that the patient is truly therapeutic, and the patient's INR should be ≥2.0 for 24 hours before heparin (or fondaparinux) is discontinued. Since the half-lives of these clotting factors are 40 hours (factor X) and 72 hours (factor II), the 5-day overlap of VKAs with heparin is necessary to ensure a therapeutic reduction in these clotting factors.

The next important question is: How long should anticoagulation be continued? Essentially all studies that have addressed the question of duration of anticoagulation have shown that the longer the anticoagulation is continued, the lower the risk of recurrence. This always must be balanced by the increased risk of bleeding.

Duration of anticoagulation

Four weeks versus three months

One of the early studies was performed by Levine et al.[7,8] when they randomized 406 patients with venographically proven proximal DVT to either

Table 7.2 ACCP recommendations for the initial treatment of acute DVT

Recommendation	Grade
Short-term treatment with LMWH.	1B
Shorter-term intravenous UFH.	1B
Short-term monitored subcutaneous UFH.	1B
Short-term fixed-dose subcutaneous UFH.	1B
Short-term subcutaneous fondaparinux.	1B
LMWH is recommended over UFH.	2C
For patients with high clinical suspicion of acute DVT, parenteral anticoagulation is recommended while awaiting diagnostic tests.	2C
For patients with an intermediate (or low) clinical suspicion of acute VTE, parenteral anticoagulation is not recommended while awaiting the results of diagnostic tests.	2C

Source: Data from Kearon C, Akl EA, Comerota AJ, et al., *Chest* 2012; 141:e419S–e494S.

Note: DVT, deep venous thrombosis; INR, international normalized ratio; LMWH, low-molecular-weight heparin; UFH, unfractionated heparin; VTE, venous thromboembolism.

4 weeks or 3 months of anticoagulation. At the completion of 4 weeks, all patients underwent impedance plethysmography (IPG), which is a physiologic study designed to detect venous outflow obstruction. If the IPG demonstrated venous outflow obstruction (assumed to be caused by persistent thrombus), patients were continued on anticoagulation for another 8 weeks. If the IPG was normal, patients were randomized to either placebo or continued anticoagulation for 8 weeks. Recurrence rates at 8 weeks were 8.6% in the placebo group versus 0.9% in the anticoagulation group ($p = .009$). At 11 months, recurrence rates were 11.5% versus 6% ($p = .3$) in the placebo and anticoagulation groups, respectively. Therefore, Levine not only demonstrated that 3 months was better than 4 weeks, but also that once anticoagulation was discontinued, recurrence rates were appreciable.

Six weeks versus six months

Schulman et al.[9] evaluated a longer duration of anticoagulation when randomizing 900 patients with a first episode of VTE to either 6 weeks or 6 months of oral anticoagulation. Their endpoints were recurrent VTE at 2 years or major bleeding. Recurrence occurred in 18.1% of patients receiving 6 weeks of anticoagulation compared with 9.5% of patients receiving 6 months of anticoagulation

(OR 2.1; $p < .001$). There was no difference in major bleeding between the groups.

Three months versus indefinite

Kearon and colleagues[10] addressed the issue of indefinite anticoagulation in patients with idiopathic VTE. They randomized patients to either 3 months or indefinite anticoagulation. The data and safety monitoring committee for the study stopped the trial at the interim analysis since recurrence occurred in 24% of the patients treated for 3 months versus 1.3% in patients receiving indefinite anticoagulation. The mean duration of anticoagulation in the indefinite group at the time of the analysis was over 1 year. The extended therapy group demonstrated a 95% relative risk reduction in recurrence ($p < .001$). There were no major bleeding episodes in the short-duration anticoagulation group versus 3.8% in the indefinite anticoagulation group ($p = .09$).

Indefinite subtherapeutic anticoagulation versus placebo

Ridker et al.[11] hypothesized that following a 3- to 6-month course of therapeutic anticoagulation, low-dose subtherapeutic anticoagulation would be safer and more effective than no therapy. They then randomized patients with VTE to subtherapeutic anticoagulation to a target INR of 1.5 to 2.0 versus placebo after a 3- to 6-month course of therapeutic anticoagulation. A total of 14.6% in the placebo group developed a recurrence versus 5.5% in the warfarin group (relative risk reduction [RRR] 62%; $p < .001$). There was no difference in major bleeding or death between the groups; however, when a composite endpoint of recurrent DVT and death was analyzed, 16.2% was observed with placebo versus 8.6% with warfarin (RRR 48%; $p = .01$). Therefore, Ridker and colleagues found that indefinite subtherapeutic anticoagulation protected against recurrence, and the combined endpoint of recurrence plus death favored indefinite subtherapeutic anticoagulation, with no significant difference in bleeding.

Indefinite subtherapeutic versus indefinite conventional anticoagulation

Shortly thereafter, Kearon et al.[12] published their randomized blinded study comparing indefinite low-intensity anticoagulation versus indefinite conventional anticoagulation for patients with VTE. They randomized 738 patients presenting with a first-time unprovoked VTE. After 3 months of therapeutic anticoagulation, patients were randomized to low-intensity treatment with VKA to a target INR of 1.5 to 1.9 versus conventional treatment with VKA to a target INR of 2.0 to 3.0. The endpoints were recurrence, death, and major bleeding. The mean follow-up for this study was 2.4 years.

The investigators found a significantly higher recurrence rate in patients receiving subtherapeutic anticoagulation versus conventional anticoagulation (HR 2.8; $p = .03$). There was a trend toward increased mortality in patients receiving subtherapeutic anticoagulation (HR 2.1; $p = .09$). There was no difference in major bleeding.

These observations plus a careful analysis of the remaining literature led the ACCP committee to make key recommendations regarding anticoagulation for a first-time venous thromboembolic event (Table 7.3).[7]

Aspirin to prevent recurrent VTE

The potential benefit of platelet inhibition in the secondary prevention of VTE was addressed in a small trial published over 30 years ago.[13] Recently, two randomized trials, the Warfarin and Aspirin (WARFASA) study[14] and the Aspirin to Prevent Recurrent Venous Thromboembolism (ASPIRE) study,[15] randomized 1225 patients with unprovoked VTE to either aspirin or placebo. All patients completed initial treatment with heparin followed by warfarin. Both studies used an identical low-dose aspirin regimen of 100 mg daily. Both studies had similar enrollment criteria and outcome measures; therefore, it was appropriate to analyze them together (Table 7.4).

The combined results of the WARFASA and ASPIRE trials show a 32% reduction in the rate of recurrent VTE ($p = .007$). There was also a 34% reduction in the rate of major vascular events compared with placebo ($p = .002$). There was no significant increased risk of bleeding.

The authors noted that those randomized to aspirin discontinued therapy at a rate of 11.9% per year; therefore, the benefit of aspirin may be underestimated when analyzed on an intent-to-treat basis, as the data are presented in Table 7.4.

Recurrent DVT

Schulman et al.[16] then addressed the issue of patients developing recurrence after a therapeutic course of anticoagulation. They randomized 480 patients with recurrent VTE to either 6 months or indefinite anticoagulation. Subsequent recurrence occurred in 21% of patients randomized to the shorter duration of therapy compared with 3% in the indefinite group (HR 8.0; $p < .001$). Although point estimates demonstrated a mortality benefit of indefinite anticoagulation, the difference did not reach statistical significance. There were, however, more major bleeds in the indefinite group (9%) versus those treated for 6 months (3%) ($p = .0084$). These observations and others led the ACCP guideline committee to recommend long-term, indefinite treatment for patients with recurrent (unprovoked) DVT. However, the committee recommends that physicians reassess the risk-benefit of indefinite anticoagulation at periodic intervals.

Table 7.3 ACCP recommendations for duration and intensity of anticoagulation therapy for DVT/VTE

Recommendation	Grade
In patients with acute VTE treated with anticoagulation, early initiation of VKA (same day as parenteral) is recommended, and continued for a minimum of 5 days and until the INR is 2.0 or above for ≥24 hours.	1B
VKA therapy for at least 3 months is recommended over shorter therapy.	1B
VKAs should be given to a target INR of 2.0–3.0 for all treatment durations.	1B
In patients with a first unprovoked proximal DVT who have a low or moderate bleeding risk, extended anticoagulation is suggested.	2B
In patients with a first unprovoked VTE who are at high risk for bleeding, 3 months of anticoagulation over extended therapy is recommended.	2B
Patients with DVT and cancer should receive LMWH over VKAs.	2B
In patients with acute isolated calf vein thrombosis and symptoms or risk factors for extension, 3 months of anticoagulation is recommended over serial imaging.	2C
In patients with acute isolated calf vein thrombosis without symptoms or risk factors for extension, serial imaging for 2 weeks is recommended over initial anticoagulation.	2C
In patients with acute calf DVT who are managed with anticoagulation, the same duration and intensity of anticoagulation are recommended as for acute femoropopliteal or iliofemoral DVT.	1B
In patients with acute calf DVT who are managed with serial imaging:	
a. No anticoagulation is recommended if the thrombus does not extend.	1B
b. Anticoagulation is recommended if the thrombus extends but remains confined to the calf veins.	2C
c. Anticoagulation is recommended if the thrombus extends to the popliteal vein or more proximally.	1B

Source: Data from Kearon C, Akl EA, Comerota AJ, et al., *Chest* 2012; 141:e419S–e494S.

Note: ACCP, American College of Chest Physicians; DVT, deep venous thrombosis; INR, international normalized ratio; LMWH, low-molecular-weight heparin; VKA, vitamin K antagonist.

TABLE 7.4 Pooled results of the WARFASA and ASPIRE trials

Outcome	Hazard ratio (95% CI)	*p* value
Venous thromboembolism	0.68 (0.51–0.90)	.007
Major vascular events	0.66 (0.51–0.86)	.002
Clinically relevant bleeding	1.47 (0.70–3.08)	.31

Source: Bright TA, et al. Low-dose aspirin for preventing recurrent venous thrombo-embolism. *N Engl J Med* 2012; 367:1979–1987.

Note: CI, confidence interval.

DVT and malignancy

The important subset of patients with DVT and malignancy was addressed by Lee et al.[17] The issue evaluated was the best form of ongoing treatment in patients with malignancy. They randomized patients to the LMWH dalteparine or VKA and found that there was a significantly higher risk of recurrence in patients randomized to the warfarin compound versus LMWH (15.8% vs. 8%; HR 0.48; *p* = .002). These observations and the results of other studies led to the recommendations

Table 7.5 Additional ACCP key recommendations for treatment of acute DVT

Recommendation	Grade
In patients with recurrent unprovoked DVT at low/moderate risk of bleeding, extended anticoagulation is recommended.	1B/2B
In patients with recurrent unprovoked DVT at high bleeding risk, 3 months of anticoagulation is recommended.	2B
In patients with cancer, LMWH is recommended over VKAs.	2B
In patients with cancer, subsequent treatment with LMWH or VKA should continue indefinitely or until the cancer is resolved.	1C
Following initiation of anticoagulation for acute DVT, early ambulation is recommended in preference to bed rest.	2C
In patients with acute symptomatic DVT, elastic compression stockings 30–40 mmHg are recommended.	2B
In patients with acute DVT of the leg, an IVC filter is not recommended in addition to anticoagulation.	1B
In patients with acute DVT involving the popliteal vein or more proximally who have contraindication to anticoagulation, an IVC filter is recommended.	1B
In patients with acute DVT who have an IVC filter inserted because of contraindication to anticoagulation, a conventional course of anticoagulation is recommended when their bleeding risk resolves.	2B

Source: Data from Kearon C, Akl EA, Comerota AJ, et al., *Chest* 2012; 141:e419S–e494S.

Note: DVT, deep venous thrombosis; IVC, inferior vena cava; LMWH, low-molecular-weight heparin; VKA, vitamin K antagonist.

favoring LMWH in preference to VKAs for the treatment of VTE in patients with cancer (Table 7.5).

Tailoring duration of anticoagulation

A number of investigators have attempted to tailor the duration of anticoagulation according to the thrombus load and degree of residual venous obstruction within the thrombosed vein or ongoing thrombus activity. Hull et al.[18] performed a systematic review of the literature and assessed outcome of patients after treatment for acute DVT, with specific attention to initial thrombus burden. Residual venous obstruction at the time anticoagulation is discontinued, as determined by ultrasound findings, and thrombus activity, as determined by D-dimer levels, have both been used in meaningful observational and randomized studies.

Residual venous obstruction on ultrasound

Many investigators reporting persistent ultrasound abnormalities over the long term characterize these ultrasound findings as "residual thrombus." In reality, thrombus no longer exists since there is reabsorption of red cells with the evolution to a fibrous, collagen intraluminal material.

Piovella et al.[19] evaluated thrombus resolution with venous ultrasound in 283 patients with acute DVT. All patients were anticoagulated for a minimum of 3 months and 16% were treated for more than 9 months. Recurrent DVT occurred in 20 patients (7%) during 12 months of follow-up. Residual luminal obstruction on venous ultrasound was the only predictor of recurrence. At 6 months follow-up, the odds ratio was 5.26 ($p = .007$) in those patients with residual obstruction compared with those with a normal ultrasound. Interestingly, in the cancer-free subgroup, the odds ratio for recurrence at 6 months with abnormal venous ultrasound was an impressive 11.29 (*p* = .002). These investigators showed that visual, persistent, intraluminal venous obstruction identified patients at high risk of recurrence.

Prandoni et al.[20] followed 313 patients with proximal DVT using venous ultrasound. This patient cohort was followed for a period of 6 years. Fifty-eight patients developed recurrence (18.5%). Forty-one (71%) had residual venous obstruction on ultrasound. They demonstrated that the risk of recurrence was significantly higher in patients with residual venous obstruction (hazard ratio 2.9; *p* = .001). It is interesting to note that only one-third of the recurrences occurred in the index leg with venous obstruction, and 43% occurred in the contralateral leg, with 24% of patients presenting with PE.[20,21]

Randomized trials

Prandoni and his group[22] tested the hypothesis that extending anticoagulation in patients with residual venous obstruction would reduce recurrence rates by performing a randomized trial. They compared the administration of a conventional fixed duration of oral anticoagulation with adjusting the duration of anticoagulation in patients with residual venous obstruction on ultrasound.

A total of 538 consecutive outpatients with a first episode of acute proximal DVT were studied following completion of a 3-month period of anticoagulation. This study sample included patients with both secondary DVT and those with unprovoked DVT. Patients were stratified according to etiology. Patients received a fixed duration of anticoagulation (no further anticoagulation for secondary thrombosis and an extra 3 months for unprovoked thrombosis) or a flexible duration of anticoagulation, which was ultrasound guided. Patients received no further anticoagulation if the veins were normal on ultrasound. Anticoagulation was continued for all other patients for up to 9 months for secondary DVT and up to 21 months for unprovoked DVT.

Results demonstrated that 17.2% of the patients randomized to fixed-duration anticoagulation developed recurrence versus 11.9% in those randomized to flexible-duration anticoagulation. It appeared that patients with unprovoked DVT enjoyed the greatest benefit by adjusting the duration of anticoagulation according to ultrasound findings, as their adjusted hazard ratio was 0.61 compared with 0.81 for those with secondary DVT (Figure 7.1).

Siragusa et al.[23] randomized 180 patients with residual thrombosis on ultrasound after 3 months of therapeutic anticoagulation into either 9 additional months of anticoagulant therapy or no further treatment. All patients who had normal

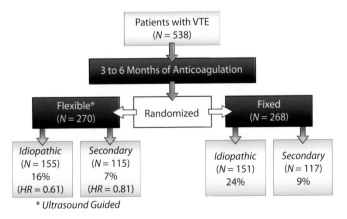

Figure 7.1 Recurrence rates in patients with VTE receiving fixed duration of anticoagulation versus flexible (extended) duration of anticoagulation based on venous ultrasound. (Data from Prandoni P, et al., *Ann Intern Med* 2009; 150:577–585.)

venous ultrasound had their anticoagulation discontinued. Follow-up was for a period of 2 years after the index event. In the group of patients with normal ultrasound, only one (1.3%) developed a recurrence. In patients with abnormal venous ultrasound examinations, 19.3% who continued on anticoagulation developed recurrence, and 27.2% in those who discontinued anticoagulation developed recurrence.

Both Siragusa et al.[23] and Prandoni et al.[22] showed that assessment of residual venous obstruction by ultrasound improves the identification of patients who are highest risk for recurrence, allowing decisions on extending anticoagulation in that group to reduce future recurrent thrombotic events.

Thrombus activity: D-dimer

D-dimer is an indicator of coagulation activation and fibrinolysis. D-dimer levels increase when complex fibrin (fibrin stabilized by factor XIIIa) is broken down by plasmin. In population-based studies, D-dimer levels positively correlated to the occurrence of a future first thrombotic event. [24]

Palareti et al.[25] hypothesized that D-dimer levels would be predictive of recurrent venous thromboembolic events in subjects with a previous unprovoked DVT or PE. These investigators prospectively followed 599 patients who were treated for either DVT or PE. One month after oral anticoagulants were withdrawn, patients had their D-dimer levels drawn and were screened for an inherited thrombophilia. Recurrent thromboembolic events occurred in 58 subjects (9.7%). Elevated D-dimer levels were associated with higher rates of subsequent recurrence in all subjects, especially those with an unprovoked venous thromboembolic event (hazard ratio 2.43). In those with a thrombophilia, the hazard ratio was 8.34. The negative predictive values of a normal D-dimer were 93% and 96% in subjects with unprovoked event or with thrombophilia, respectively. These important observations clarify that the risk of recurrence is related to thrombus activity rather than the presence of an inherited thrombophilia.

Eichinger et al.[26] also prospectively evaluated the link between recurrent VTE and D-dimer levels after oral anticoagulants were discontinued.

They prospectively followed 610 patients who received a minimum 3-month course of oral anticoagulation after an initial spontaneous venous thromboembolic event. D-dimer levels were measured 1 month after anticoagulation was discontinued.

Thirteen percent of the 610 patients had a recurrent event at a mean of 38 months of follow-up. Patients with recurrent VTE had a significantly higher D-dimer level compared to those with no recurrence ($p = .01$). In patients with a D-dimer level less than 250 ng/mL, the risk of recurrence at 2 years was 3.7% compared to 11.5% ($p = .001$) among patients with higher D-dimer levels.

Randomized trial

Palareti et al.[27] for the PROLONG investigators tested the hypothesis that D-dimer could be used to determine a more proper duration of anticoagulation for patients with VTE. They performed D-dimer testing 1 month after discontinuation of anticoagulation in patients with a first-time unprovoked proximal DVT or PE who had received VKA for a minimum of 3 months. Patients with normal D-dimer levels took no further anticoagulation. Patients with abnormal D-dimer levels were randomized to continue anticoagulation versus no further anticoagulation.

Fifteen percent of the patients with an abnormal D-dimer level who were not protected with anticoagulation developed recurrence within 1.4 years compared to only 2.9% who had abnormal D-dimer levels but who had resumed anticoagulation. This yields an adjusted hazard ratio of 4.26 ($p = .02$). The recurrence rate was 6.2% in patients with normal D-dimer levels who did not receive ongoing anticoagulation. The cumulative incidence for the main outcome of recurrence by treatment group is shown in Figure 7.2.

This trial clearly demonstrates that patients with increased thrombus activity manifested by elevated D-dimer levels significantly benefit from ongoing anticoagulation. Patients with normal D-dimer levels continue to have an appreciable risk of recurrence (6.2% at 18 months); therefore, proper management for this cohort of patients has not yet been established.

Cosmi et al.[28] performed a post hoc analysis of the PROLONG study, integrating the venous ultrasound results with D-dimer results to determine

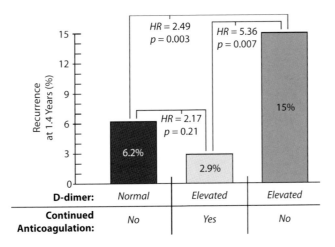

Figure 7.2 Cumulative recurrent rates by treatment group: D-dimer level and anticoagulation. (Data from Palareti G, et al., *N Engl J Med* 2006; 355:1780–1789.)

if combining these two measures will improve the predictive capability of recurrence. These investigators found that recurrence occurred in 19% of patients with abnormal D-dimer levels who did not resume anticoagulation and 10% in subjects with normal D-dimer levels ($p = .02$). Recurrences were similar in subjects with residual venous obstruction on venous ultrasound (11%) and those without (13%). Interestingly, they found that recurrent DVT rates were similar for normal D-dimer patients, with or without residual venous obstruction, and for abnormal D-dimer patients, with or without residual venous obstruction.

The inconsistency in recurrence rates observed between studies may be due to differences in patient sample as well as the potentially small sample size. Differences in the technique and interpretation of the venous ultrasound also need to be considered. Unquestionably, more work will be done in this area; however, the observations to date should help clinicians more properly identify those patients at risk of recurrence.

The ACCP committee has not made any recommendation regarding use of venous ultrasound or D-dimer to assist in modifying the duration of anticoagulation for acute DVT. However, based upon the available literature and the results of randomized trials, a suggested algorithm for establishing the appropriate duration of anticoagulation is presented in Figure 7.3 and is used by this author.

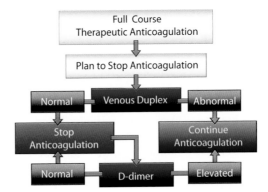

Figure 7.3 Suggested algorithm for managing the duration of anticoagulation in patients with a first episode of DVT.

Ambulation and compression

Physicians are increasingly recognizing the benefit of leg compression and early ambulation in patients with acute DVT. There are five randomized trials[29–33] and three observational studies[34–36] evaluating early ambulation versus bed rest in patients with acute DVT. The majority of the ambulated patients also had compression applied from the base of the toes to at least the knee, and most to the thigh level. Early ambulation with compression after the initiation of anticoagulation resulted in more rapid resolution of pain and swelling and less postthrombotic morbidity, with no increased risk of PE. As a result, the ACCP has recommended early ambulation in preference to initial bed rest.

The continued use of effective elastic compression stockings at a 30 to 40 mmHg ankle-gradient pressure was clearly shown in two randomized trials. Brandjes et al.[37] and Prandoni et al.[38] demonstrated a 51% to 55% relative risk reduction in postthrombotic syndrome in patients who wore well-fit 30–40 mmHg elastic compression stockings versus those who did not wear compression ($p < .01$). Therefore, elastic compression stockings with an ankle gradient of 30 to 40 mmHg of pressure are recommended for ongoing treatment of patients with acute DVT. Of course, if early thrombus resolution occurs and the patient has no swelling, and noninvasive studies demonstrate patent veins with normal valve function, long-term compression is not required.

REFERENCES

1. Barritt DW, Jordan SC. Anticoagulant drugs in the treatment of pulmonary embolism: a controlled trial. *Lancet* 1960; 1:1309–1312.
2. Brandjes DP, Heijboer H, Buller HR, de Rijk M, Jagt H, ten Cate JW. Acenocoumarol and heparin compared with acenocoumarol alone in the initial treatment of proximal-vein thrombosis. *N Engl J Med* 1992; 327:1485–1489.
3. Hull RD, Raskob GE, Hirsh J, et al. Continuous intravenous heparin compared with intermittent subcutaneous heparin in the initial treatment of proximal-vein thrombosis. *N Engl J Med* 1986; 315:1109–1114.
4. Hull RD, Raskob GE, Brant RF, Pineo GF, Valentine KA. Relation between the time to achieve the lower limit of the APTT therapeutic range and recurrent venous thromboembolism during heparin treatment for deep vein thrombosis. *Arch Intern Med* 1997; 157:2562–2568.
5. Van Dongen CJ, van den Belt AG, Prins MH, Lensing AW. Fixed dose subcutaneous low molecular weight heparins versus adjusted dose unfractionated heparin for venous thromboembolism. *Cochrane Database Syst Rev* 2004;CD001100.
6. Othieno R, Abu AM, Okpo E. Home versus in-patient treatment for deep vein thrombosis. *Cochrane Database Syst Rev* 2007; CD003076.
7. Kearon C, Akl EA, Comerota AJ, et al. Antithrombotic therapy for VTE disease: Antithrombotic Therapy and Prevention of Thrombosis, 9th ed: American College of Chest Physicians Evidence-Based Clinical Practice Guidelines. *Chest* 2012; 141:e419S–e494S.
8. Levine MN, Hirsh J, Gent M, et al. Optimal duration of oral anticoagulant therapy: a randomized trial comparing four weeks with three months of warfarin in patients with proximal deep vein thrombosis. *Thromb Haemost* 1995; 74:606–611.
9. Schulman S, Rhedin AS, Lindmarker P, et al. A comparison of six weeks with six months of oral anticoagulant therapy after a first episode of venous thromboembolism. Duration of Anticoagulation Trial Study Group. *N Engl J Med* 1995; 332:1661–1665.
10. Kearon C, Gent M, Hirsh J, et al. A comparison of three months of anticoagulation with extended anticoagulation for a first episode of idiopathic venous thromboembolism. *N Engl J Med* 1999; 340:901–907.
11. Ridker PM, Goldhaber SZ, Danielson E, et al. Long-term, low-intensity warfarin therapy for the prevention of recurrent venous thromboembolism. *N Engl J Med* 2003; 348:1425–1434.
12. Kearon C, Ginsberg JS, Kovacs MJ, et al. Comparison of low-intensity warfarin therapy with conventional-intensity warfarin therapy for long-term prevention of recurrent venous thromboembolism. *N Engl J Med* 2003; 349:631–639.
13. Steele P. Trial of dipyridamole-aspirin in recurring venous thrombosis. *Lancet* 1980; 2:1328–1329.
14. Becattini C, Agnelli GA, Schenone A, et al. Aspirin for preventing the recurrence of venous thromboembolism. *N Engl J Med* 2012; 366:1959–1967.
15. Brighton TA, Eikelboom JW, Mann K, et al. Low-dose aspirin for preventing recurrent

venous thromboembolism. *N Engl J Med* 2012; 367:1979–1987.

16. Schulman S, Granqvist S, Holmstrom M, et al. The duration of oral anticoagulant therapy after a second episode of venous thromboembolism. The Duration of Anticoagulation Trial Study Group. *N Engl J Med* 1997; 336:393–398.

17. Lee AY, Levine MN, Baker RI, et al. Low-molecular-weight heparin versus a coumarin for the prevention of recurrent venous thromboembolism in patients with cancer. *N Engl J Med* 2003; 349:146–153.

18. Hull RD, Marder VJ, Mah AF, Biel RK, Brant RF. Quantitative assessment of thrombus burden predicts the outcome of treatment for venous thrombosis: a systematic review. *Am J Med* 2005; 118:456–464.

19. Piovella F, Crippa L, Barone M, et al. Normalization rates of compression ultrasonography in patients with a first episode of deep vein thrombosis of the lower limbs: association with recurrence and new thrombosis. *Haematologica* 2002; 87:515–522.

20. Prandoni P. Risk factors of recurrent venous thromboembolism: the role of residual vein thrombosis. *Pathophysiol Haemost Thromb* 2003; 33:351–353.

21. Prandoni P, Lensing AW, Prins MH, et al. Residual venous thrombosis as a predictive factor of recurrent venous thromboembolism. *Ann Intern Med* 2002; 137:955–960.

22. Prandoni P, Prins MH, Lensing AW, et al. Residual thrombosis on ultrasonography to guide the duration of anticoagulation in patients with deep venous thrombosis: a randomized trial. *Ann Intern Med* 2009; 150:577–585.

23. Siragusa S, Malato A, Anastasio R, et al. Residual vein thrombosis to establish duration of anticoagulation after a first episode of deep vein thrombosis: the Duration of Anticoagulation based on Compression Ultrasonography (DACUS) study. *Blood* 2008; 112:511–515.

24. Cushman M, Folsom AR, Wang L, et al. Fibrin fragment D-dimer and the risk of future venous thrombosis. Blood 2003; 101:1243–1248.

25. Palareti G, Legnani C, Cosmi B, et al. Predictive value of D-dimer test for recurrent venous thromboembolism after anticoagulation withdrawal in subjects with a previous idiopathic event and in carriers of congenital thrombophilia. *Circulation* 2003; 108:313–318.

26. Eichinger S, Minar E, Bialonczyk C, et al. D-dimer levels and risk of recurrent venous thromboembolism. *JAMA* 2003; 290:1071–1074.

27. Palareti G, Cosmi B, Legnani C, et al. D-dimer testing to determine the duration of anticoagulation therapy. *N Engl J Med* 2006; 355:1780–1789.

28. Cosmi B, Legnani C, Iorio A, et al. Residual venous obstruction, alone and in combination with D-dimer, as a risk factor for recurrence after anticoagulation withdrawal following a first idiopathic deep vein thrombosis in the PROLONG study. *Eur J Vasc Endovasc Surg* 2010; 39:356–365.

29. Aschwanden M, Labs KH, Engel H, et al. Acute deep vein thrombosis: early mobilization does not increase the frequency of pulmonary embolism. *Thromb Haemost* 2001; 85:42–46.

30. Blattler W, Partsch H. Leg compression and ambulation is better than bed rest for the treatment of acute deep venous thrombosis. *Int Angiol* 2003; 22:393–400.

31. Junger M, Diehm C, Storiko H, et al. Mobilization versus immobilization in the treatment of acute proximal deep venous thrombosis: a prospective, randomized, open, multicentre trial. *Curr Med Res Opin* 2006; 22:593–602.

32. Partsch H, Blattler W. Compression and walking versus bed rest in the treatment of proximal deep venous thrombosis with low molecular weight heparin. *J Vasc Surg* 2000; 32:861–869.

33. Schellong SM, Schwarz T, Kropp J, Prescher Y, Beuthien-Baumann B, Daniel WG. Bed rest in deep vein thrombosis and the incidence of scintigraphic pulmonary embolism. *Thromb Haemost* 1999; 82(Suppl 1):127–129.

34. Partsch H, Kaulich M, Mayer W. Immediate mobilisation in acute vein thrombosis

reduces post-thrombotic syndrome. *Int Angiol* 2004; 23:206–212.

35. Partsch H. Therapy of deep vein thrombosis with low molecular weight heparin, leg compression and immediate ambulation. *Vasa* 2001; 30:195–204.

36. Trujillo-Santos J, Perea-Milla E, Jimenez-Puente A, et al. Bed rest or ambulation in the initial treatment of patients with acute deep vein thrombosis or pulmonary embolism: findings from the RIETE registry. *Chest* 2005; 127:1631–1636.

37. Brandjes DP, Buller HR, Heijboer H, et al. Randomised trial of effect of compression stockings in patients with symptomatic proximal-vein thrombosis. *Lancet* 1997; 349:759–762.

38. Prandoni P, Lensing AW, Prins MH, et al. Below-knee elastic compression stockings to prevent the post-thrombotic syndrome: a randomized, controlled trial. *Ann Intern Med* 2004; 141:249–256.

8

Strategy of thrombus removal

Background

A large body of evidence indicates that early elimination of thrombus prevents or reduces post-thrombotic morbidity. This is especially true in patients with iliofemoral deep vein thrombosis (DVT). Considering that the common femoral vein, external iliac vein, and common iliac vein are a single channel responsible for the entire venous drainage from the lower extremity, occlusion of the iliofemoral system leads to severe venous hypertension at the time of the acute event[1] and persistently high venous pressures chronically.[2] Early removal of the thrombus from the iliofemoral system restores venous (compartment) pressures to normal[1]; therefore, it would be anticipated that eliminating acute outflow obstruction would substantially improve long-term results. Every randomized trial to date and essentially all comparative studies assessing the value of thrombus removal in patients with iliofemoral DVT have demonstrated benefit.

The 2008 American College of Chest Physicians (ACCP) guidelines include suggestions for early thrombus removal (Table 8.1).[3] These suggestions for patient care were reinforced by the American Heart Association (AHA) and American College of Cardiology (ACC) guidelines.[4] Recognizing that extensive venous thrombosis is associated with severe long-term postthrombotic morbidity and that evidence supports the use of venous thrombectomy and catheter-directed thrombolysis (CDT), the authors suggested the use of these treatments for iliofemoral DVT. The authors went on to suggest that systemic thrombolytic therapy be considered in communities in which venous thrombectomy

or catheter-directed techniques are not available. However, since only a small portion of the systemically delivered plasminogen activator will contact the occlusive thrombus, results of systemic thrombolysis will not be nearly as efficacious as catheter-directed intrathrombus pharmacomechanical techniques. Furthermore, bleeding complications are likely to be substantially higher because higher doses of plasminogen activator are used that produce a sustained systemic lytic state.[5]

Rationale for thrombus removal

The major reason to adopt a strategy of thrombus removal is the severe morbidity associated with the postthrombotic syndrome resulting from extensive DVT, especially iliofemoral DVT. Studies have shown that patients with postthrombotic syndrome have a significant reduction in their quality of life.[6-9] The severity of acute DVT, especially iliofemoral DVT, is predictive of postthrombotic morbidity.[9] Iliofemoral DVT is a clinically important subset of patients with acute DVT in that their postthrombotic morbidity is particularly severe.[6-8] Patients with iliofemoral DVT who are treated with anticoagulation alone face markedly elevated ambulatory venous pressures, which results in objective findings of venous insufficiency in over 90% of patients. Forty percent will have symptoms of venous claudication,[8] and up to 15% will develop venous ulcers within 5 years.[7] Essentially all of these patients will have a marked reduction in their quality of life. The consistent evidence extending from animal experimentation,[10,11] observational

Table 8.1 Key ACCP recommendations for patients with iliofemoral DVT

Recommendations	Grade
In selected patients (symptoms < 7 days, good functional status, life expectancy > 1 year), operative venous thrombectomy is suggested to reduce acute symptoms and postthrombotic morbidity.	2B
In patients who undergo operative venous thrombectomy, it is recommended that the same duration and intensity of anticoagulation therapy be prescribed as for comparable patients who did not undergo venous thrombectomy.	1C
In selected patients with iliofemoral DVT (symptoms < 14 days, good functional status, life expectancy > 1 year) who have a low risk of bleeding, catheter-directed thrombolysis is suggested to reduce acute symptoms and postthrombotic morbidity.	2B
Following successful catheter-directed thrombolysis, correction of underlying venous lesions using balloon angioplasty and stenting is suggested.	2C
Pharmacomechanical thrombolysis is suggested in preference to catheter-directed thrombolysis to shorten treatment time.	2C
Following successful catheter-directed thrombolysis, the same duration and intensity of anticoagulation therapy should be prescribed as for comparable patients who did not undergo catheter-directed thrombolysis.	1C

Source: Data from Kearon C, et al., *Chest* 2008; 133:454S–545S.

Note: ACCP, American College of Chest Physicians; DVT, deep venous thrombosis.

studies,[12–14] natural history studies,[12–14] and randomized trials[15–17] shows that a strategy of thrombus removal is the preferred management option for iliofemoral DVT and offers the patient the best long-term outcome.

Postthrombotic morbidity of iliofemoral DVT

Postthrombotic chronic venous disease results from ambulatory venous hypertension, defined as elevated venous pressure during exercise.[18,19] Increases in ambulatory venous pressure are linearly correlated with the clinical progression of venous disease as described by the clinical class of CEAP (clinical, etiologic, anatomic, pathophysiologic),[20] from C_1 to C_4. Some patients will progress from C_4 to develop skin breakdown (C_6), whereas others will not. This progression is due to changes in the microcirculation as opposed to further increases in ambulatory venous pressure.[21]

The anatomic components causing ambulatory venous hypertension are venous valvular incompetence and luminal obstruction. While calf muscle pump function is also an important component of ambulatory venous pressure, it is predominantly linked to the mobility of the ankle joint, which cannot be necessarily altered by treatment options for acute DVT. However, ankle motion will deteriorate if ambulation is painful and the ankle is encompassed by significant edema. Ankle joint mobility promotes good calf muscle pump function, whereas restricted range of motion with edema reduces mobility. The most severe postthrombotic morbidity is associated with the highest venous pressures, which occur in patients who have both valvular incompetence and luminal venous obstruction.[14,18] Although venous valve function is reliably assessed with ultrasound and can be quantified by accurately recording valve closure time, present techniques are not capable of assessing venous obstruction and its contribution to the pathologic venous hemodynamics leading to postthrombotic morbidity.

Figure 8.1 illustrates the difficulty in identifying even extensive venous obstruction, either hemodynamically or radiologically. Neither ascending phlebography, which was performed and interpreted by a skilled radiologist, nor a maximal venous outflow test, performed in an accredited vascular laboratory using a standardized

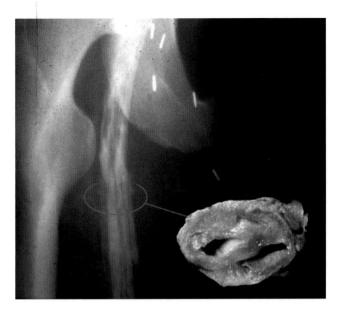

Figure 8.1 The inability to identify obstruction as part of the pathophysiology of chronic venous disease is illustrated in this patient, who was treated with anticoagulation alone for iliofemoral DVT 10 years earlier. His severe postthrombotic syndrome required multiple hospitalizations for venous ulceration. An ascending phlebogram showed recanalization of the iliofemoral venous system, and the radiological interpretation was that there was "no obstruction" of the deep venous system and a 3-second maximal venous outflow test was "normal." A "classic Linton procedure" was performed showing (inset) the cross section of the femoral vein at the corresponding location on the phlebogram, just below the profunda femoris vein.

technique, identified obstruction as part of the patient's postthrombotic pathophysiology. A cross section of the femoral vein removed during a classic Linton procedure performed the day following the venogram and impedance plethysmography clearly shows the substantial degree of obstruction remaining after anticoagulation for iliofemoral DVT. The recanalization channels that formed through what was once occlusive thrombus allowed some venous return; however, a large proportion of the luminal surface area remained obstructed. Unfortunately, the magnitude of obstruction is not appreciated radiologically or physiologically by current techniques.

There is a basic inconsistency in the way noninvasive testing is performed to assess whether venous obstruction exists. The pathophysiology of chronic venous disease is defined and quantified in the upright exercising patient, whereas the evaluation of obstruction to venous return is performed in the resting supine patient with his or her leg elevated. It is evident that venous hemodynamics are adversely affected long before imaging techniques

can detect obstruction. The inability to quantitate venous obstruction has led physicians to underappreciate its contribution to postthrombotic pathophysiology. Luminal venous obstruction causes the most severe postthrombotic syndrome. Therefore, treatment strategies for thrombus removal should be considered during the initial encounter with the patient at the time of his or her acute DVT. If successful, thrombus removal eliminates obstruction as part of the long-term pathophysiology and will significantly improve patient outcome. Furthermore, successful thrombus removal is likely to preserve valve function.

On the other hand, anticoagulation for occlusive iliofemoral DVT results in severe long-term postthrombotic venous outflow obstruction. Management of patients with chronic iliofemoral venous obstruction can be successful with endovenectomy of the chronically scarred common femoral vein and transluminal recanalization of the chronically occluded iliac veins[22] (see Chapter 11). While disobliteration of the chronically occluded iliofemoral venous system significantly improves the quality of life of these patients, the magnitude of benefit is not comparable to what can be achieved by early and complete thrombus removal.

Experimental observations in canine models of acute DVT have shown that successful thrombolysis preserves endothelial function and valve competence.[10,11] These observations translate into improved clinical outcomes when put into the perspective of natural history studies of acute DVT treated with anticoagulation alone. Investigators have found that distal valve incompetence occurs in patients with persistent proximal venous obstruction, even when the distal veins were not initially involved with thrombus.[23] However, if spontaneous lysis occurs early, generally within 90 days, valve function was found to be preserved in the majority of patients.[12] These investigators confirmed that the combination of valvular incompetence and venous obstruction was associated with the most severe postthrombotic morbidity.[13] It is logical that successful elimination of acute venous thrombus eliminates luminal obstruction, restores vein patency, and increases the likelihood that normal valve function will be preserved.

There is a misconception that acute thrombus rapidly destroys the venous valves. As mentioned earlier, Sevitt, in his classic studies of acute DVT,[24,25] demonstrated that venous clot is not attached to the valve cusp in the majority of cases. The clot is fixed to the vein wall (but not the valve cusp), most likely due to inherent physiologic differences in the endothelium of the vein wall compared to the endothelium of the valve cusp[26] (see Chapter 1).

In light of these observations, it is understandable that clot resolution restores vein patency and is capable of preserving valve function, since in most instances the clot was not physically attached to the valve leaflet. If, however, the thrombus encompassing the valve is not lysed and allowed to remain in the vein, when the thrombus retracts, the entrapped vein valve will be retracted as part of the fibrous resolution of the acute clot, resulting in relative venous obstruction and valve incompetence.

Acceptance of thrombus removal

Strategies of thrombus removal have not been widely accepted by the medical community due to the lack of randomized trials, absence of recommendations from national and international guideline committees, and a generally poor understanding of postthrombotic morbidity and how it can be avoided.

Focusing on outdated outcome information from nonrandomized trials has misled physicians into believing that venous thrombectomy is inadequate treatment for iliofemoral DVT. Critics of venous thrombectomy refer to data reported over 45 years ago, when vascular surgical procedures were crude and vascular surgery as a recognized specialty did not exist. Furthermore, the appreciation of therapeutic anticoagulation and the morbidity of recurrent DVT were not yet recognized. A more grievous oversight was overlooking a contemporary randomized trial of venous thrombectomy versus anticoagulation that reported 6-month, 5-year, and 10-year follow-ups,[15–17] which conflicted with the committee's opinion that venous thrombectomy was ineffective. The multicenter randomized trial reported that patients undergoing venous thrombectomy had improved iliac vein patency, lower venous pressures, less edema, and fewer postthrombotic symptoms than did patients receiving anticoagulation alone (all $p < .05$). The Scandinavian investigators reported that operated patients were more likely to retain venous valve function in their femoropopliteal segment than patients who were treated with anticoagulation alone. This observation is consistent with that reported by Killewich and coauthors,[23] who demonstrated that persistent proximal obstruction led to distal valve incompetence, even when the distal veins were not initially involved with thrombus. Furthermore, resolution of proximal thrombus preserved distal valve function.

An ever-increasing body of evidence suggests that catheter-based techniques are beneficial for patients with acute proximal DVT, especially in patients with iliofemoral DVT. Case-controlled studies have shown significantly improved quality of life in patients treated with catheter-directed thrombolysis versus anticoagulation alone for iliofemoral DVT.[9] A randomized trial demonstrated significantly improved venous patency and preservation of valvular function in patients receiving catheter-directed thrombolysis compared with anticoagulation alone.[27] This information, which was available at the time, was also overlooked by previous guideline writing committees.[28] There is little argument that large randomized trial data are desired for definitive treatment recommendations. However, absent data from large randomized trials, the substantial body of observational, natural history, clinical, case-controlled, and smaller randomized trial evidence supports a strategy of thrombus removal, especially in patients with iliofemoral DVT.

Treatment options for thrombus removal

Contemporary venous thrombectomy should be available for all patients in medical centers staffed by vascular surgeons. Venous thrombectomy uses standard techniques that follow the basic principles of good vascular surgery.[29] There are few contraindications to operative thrombectomy short of old thrombus, which adheres to the vein wall and cannot be removed. The goal of venous thrombectomy is to remove the iliofemoral and infrainguinal thrombus and restore unobstructed venous return to the vena cava. It is important to recognize the full extent of thrombosis preoperatively and to have good imaging intraoperatively to successfully complete a well-planned procedure.

Catheter-directed thrombolysis or *pharmacomechanical thrombolysis* is the preferred treatment option for most patients who have no absolute contraindication to thrombolytic therapy. Adjunctive mechanical techniques are increasingly popular and tend to shorten treatment time, reduce lytic dose, and improve the overall volume of thrombus removed.

Contemporary venous thrombectomy

Good short- and long-term outcomes have been observed following contemporary venous thrombectomy for iliofemoral DVT. The procedure is associated with relatively few complications. In a report of 230 patients undergoing venous thrombectomy, only one operative death occurred and no fatal pulmonary embolisms (PEs) were observed.[30] The long-term benefits of venous thrombectomy are dependent upon its ability to

restore patency to the proximal venous system. Once thrombus is removed, it is likely that valve function will be preserved. Both patency and preservation of valve function are influenced by the initial technical success and the avoidance of recurrent thrombosis. Therefore, attention to operative detail, removal of all thrombus, correction of underlying lesions, and avoidance of rethrombosis by maintenance of therapeutic anticoagulation postoperatively are crucial.

The Scandinavian investigators performed a randomized trial of operative venous thrombectomy versus anticoagulation alone in patients with iliofemoral venous thrombosis.[15-17] Patients had careful follow-up with venous imaging and physiologic measurements. Six-month, 5-year, and 10-year results showed that patients randomized to venous thrombectomy had improved patency ($p < .05$), lower venous pressure ($p < .05$), less leg edema ($p < .05$), and fewer postthrombotic symptoms ($p < .05$) than patients treated with anticoagulation alone.

Technique of venous thrombectomy

A brief overview of the important points of contemporary venous thrombectomy is provided in Table 8.2. Operative venous thrombectomy follows the principles of good basic vascular surgical technique: removing all thrombus, restoring unobstructed outflow from the iliofemoral venous segment, providing unobstructed inflow from the infrainguinal venous segment (to the common femoral vein), correcting underlying venous lesions (especially in the iliofemoral segment), and preventing rethrombosis by constructing an arteriovenous fistula (AVF) and ensuring effective anticoagulation.

Preoperative care

Preoperative anticoagulation is frequently initiated with unfractionated heparin (UFH) because it has a short half-life and can be controlled more easily than low-molecular-weight heparin (LMWH) or fondaparinux. The full extent of thrombus both distally and proximally should be identified.

Venal caval filters are not routinely used, except in patients who have nonocclusive thrombus in their vena cava. Permanent or optional filters and proximal balloon occlusion of the vena cava

Table 8.2 Overview of technique of contemporary venous thrombectomy

1. Identify etiology of extensive venous thromboembolic process
    a. Complete thrombophilia evaluation
    b. Rapid CT scan of chest, abdomen, pelvis, and head
2. Define full extent of thrombus
    a. Venous duplex examination
    b. Contralateral iliocavagram, MRV, or spiral CT
3. Prevent pulmonary embolism (numerous techniques)
    a. Anticoagulation
    b. Vena caval filter (if nonocclusive caval clot)
    c. Balloon occlusion of vena cava during thrombectomy
    d. Positive end-expiratory pressure during thrombectomy
4. Perform complete thrombectomy
    a. Iliofemoral (vena cava) thrombectomy
    b. Infrainguinal venous thrombectomy (if required)
5. Ensure unobstructed venous inflow to and outflow from thrombectomized iliofemoral venous system
    a. Infrainguinal venous thrombectomy (if required)
    b. Correct iliac vein stenosis (if present)
    c. Document with completion phlebogram
6. Prevent recurrent thrombosis
    a. Arteriovenous fistula
    b. Continuous therapeutic anticoagulation
    c. Catheter-directed postoperative anticoagulation (if infrainguinal venous thrombectomy is required)
    d. Extended oral anticoagulation

Note: MRV, magnetic resonance venography; CT, computerized tomography.

during thrombectomy (Figure 8.2a–d) are reasonable options for proximal protection from potential embolization of the nonocclusive thrombus.

The thrombectomy is performed under fluoroscopic guidance, filling the balloon of the venous thrombectomy catheter with contrast solution to follow the course of the catheter. The entire abdominal vena cava and pelvic venous system need to be in the fluoroscopic field. Autotransfusion devices are made available during the operation in case there is a need to return blood that is flushed from the venous system during the procedure.

Operative technique

Figure 8.3 provides an illustrative overview of the technique of infrainguinal venous thrombectomy.

General anesthesia is usually recommended for patients undergoing operative venous thrombectomy. A longitudinal inguinal incision is used to expose the common femoral vein, femoral vein, saphenofemoral junction, and profunda femoris vein(s). It is important to control all side branches in order to avoid blood loss when the venotomy is performed. A longitudinal venotomy is made in the common femoral vein to ensure access to the origin of the saphenous and profunda femoris branches.

If infrainguinal thrombus is present, the leg is elevated and compressed with a tightly wrapped rubber bandage. The foot is dorsiflexed and the calf and thigh are squeezed. If all infrainguinal thrombus is removed with these maneuvers, balloon thrombectomy of the iliofemoral system can proceed.

If the infrainguinal thrombus persists, a cutdown is performed to expose the distal posterior

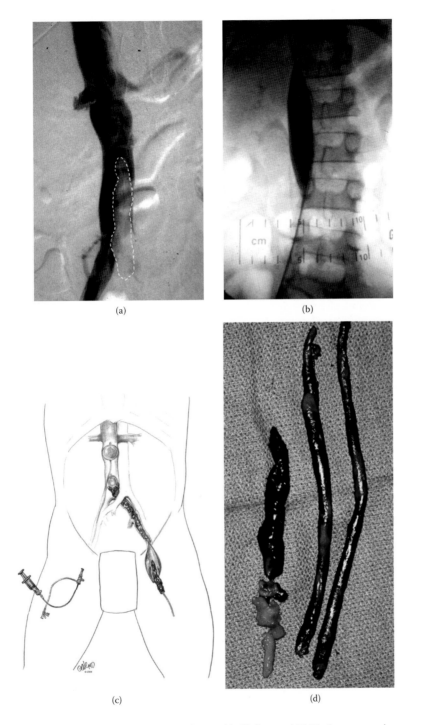

(a)

(b)

(c)

(d)

Figure 8.2 (a) Contralateral iliocavagrams in a patient with iliofemoral DVT. Cavagram shows nonocclusive thrombus extending into vena cava. Under fluoroscopy, a balloon catheter was passed proximal to the thrombus and the balloon inflated (b) to protect against embolization during venous thrombectomy. (c) Schematic of iliocaval thrombectomy with proximal balloon occlusion. (d) Specimen shows that the entire amount of thrombus was extracted. Note the more chronic platelet/fibrin thrombus that was removed from the left column iliac vein.

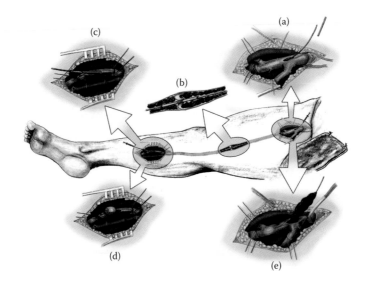

Figure 8.3 (a) The technique of infrainguinal venous thrombectomy begins with exposure of the common femoral, femoral, and profunda femoris veins, the saphenofemoral junction proximally, and the distal posterior tibial vein. A #3 Fogarty catheter is passed proximally from the distal posterior tibial vein venotomy and exits through the common femoral venotomy. A #4 Fogarty catheter is guided distally by the #3 catheter after both are placed into the silastic stem of an intravenous catheter. (b) The balloons are inflated to secure the catheter tips inside the sheath and pressure applied by a single individual to guide them distally through the thrombosed veins and venous valves. (c) The catheters and sheath exit the posterior tibial venotomy. (d) The thrombectomy catheter balloon is gently inflated as the catheter is pulled proximally (e) to exit the femoral venotomy, extracting thrombus.

tibial vein. A #3 Fogarty catheter is advanced from the distal posterior tibial vein to and through the common femoral venotomy. The silastic stem of an intravenous catheter (12 to 14 gauge) is amputated from its hub and slid halfway onto the #3 Fogarty catheter, which is now in the operative field as it has exited from the common femoral venotomy. Another balloon catheter (#4 Fogarty) is placed in the opposite end of the silastic sheath. Pressure is applied to the two balloons by a single operating surgeon to ensure that the catheters remain secure within the sheath with constant pressure in both balloons. The #4 balloon catheter is guided distally through the thrombosed venous system and easily passes through the vein valves to the level of the posterior tibial venotomy. The infrainguinal venous thrombectomy is then routinely performed in the direction of the venous valves. Passage is repeated as necessary.

Alternatively, rather than performing a cutdown on the posterior tibial vein, it can be accessed under ultrasound guidance using the micropuncture technique. A guidewire can then be advanced

to exit the common femoral venotomy and an over-the-wire thrombectomy balloon catheter can be passed distally to perform the infrainguinal venous thrombectomy.

Following infrainguinal balloon catheter thrombectomy, the infrainguinal venous system is flushed by placing a large red rubber catheter into the proximal posterior tibial vein and vigorously flushing with a heparin-saline solution via a bulb syringe to hydraulically force residual thrombus from the deep venous system (in those patients with operative exposure) (Figure 8.4). An impressive amount of thrombus is frequently flushed from the common femoral venotomy with this maneuver. Once the infrainguinal venous system is adequately cleared, a vascular clamp is gently applied below the femoral venotomy and the infrainguinal venous system is filled with a dilute plasminogen activator solution consisting of approximately 4 to 6 mg of recombinant tissue plasminogen activator (rt-PA) in 200 mL of saline. This maneuver is intended for the rt-PA to bind to fibrin-bound plasminogen in

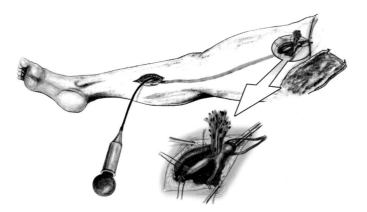

Figure 8.4 After balloon catheter thrombectomy, the venous system is flushed with a large volume of a heparin-saline solution.

residual thrombus to promote further clot dissolution; however, this minimal dose will not result in a systemic lytic effect. If the infrainguinal venous thrombectomy is not successful because of chronic disease, the femoral vein is ligated and divided below the profunda femoral vein. Patency of the profunda is ensured by direct thrombectomy if necessary.

Removal of the clot from the iliofemoral venous segment is then performed by passing a #8–10 venous thrombectomy balloon catheter partially into the iliac vein for several passes to remove the bulk of the thrombus before advancing the catheter into the vena cava in order to minimize resistance during thrombectomy. The proximal thrombectomy is always performed under fluoroscopic guidance with contrast solution in the balloon. This is especially important if a vena caval filter is present, there is clot in the vena cava, or resistance to catheter passage is encountered. During this part of the procedure, the anesthesiologist applies positive end-expiratory pressure to further reduce the risk for PE. If a clot is present in the vena cava, caval thrombectomy can be performed with a protective balloon catheter inflated above the thrombus as an alternative to vena caval filtration (Figure 8.2). Following completion of the iliofemoral venous thrombectomy, intraoperative phlebography/fluoroscopy is performed to evaluate for an underlying iliac vein stenosis and assess the venous drainage into the vena cava. Intravascular ultrasound is often better than phlebography for detecting iliac

vein stenosis. An underlying iliac vein stenosis is corrected by balloon angioplasty and stenting. If an iliac vein stent is used, a 12 mm diameter or larger stent is recommended for the external iliac vein and a 14 mm or larger stent for the common iliac vein.

Once the venotomy is closed, an end-to-side AVF is constructed by anastomosing the amputated end of the proximal saphenous vein or a large proximal branch of the saphenous vein to the side of the superficial femoral artery. If the saphenous vein is thrombosed, a thrombectomy is performed of the proximal vein and saphenofemoral junction prior to construction of the AVF. The AVF anastomosis should be limited to 3.5 to 4 mm in diameter to avoid a steal. A small vascular punch (3.5 mm) is used to produce an appropriately sized and shaped arteriotomy. The purpose of the AVF is to increase venous velocity but not iliofemoral venous pressure. Common femoral vein pressure is then recorded before and after the AVF is opened. An increase in pressure should not be observed when the AVF is opened. If the pressure increases, the proximal iliac vein should be reevaluated for an uncorrected residual stenosis (or obstruction) and the lesion corrected. If the pressure remains elevated, the AVF should be constricted to decrease flow and normalize pressure.

A piece of polytetrafluoroethylene or silastic is placed around the saphenous AVF and a large permanent monofilament suture (#0) is looped and clipped, with approximately 2 cm tail left in the

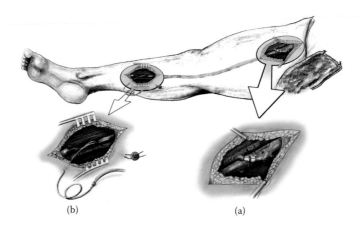

(b)   (a)

Figure 8.5 (a) Construction of an arteriovenous fistula (AVF) with a polytetrafluoroethylene (PTFE) wrap around the AVF to guide operative closure in the event it is required. (b) A small catheter (pediatric feeding tube) is placed into the proximal posterior tibial vein, entering the wound through a separate stab wound. A loop of 2-0 monofilament suture is placed around the proximal posterior tibial vein and brought out through the skin and through a sterile button. This is secured in a snug fashion when the catheter is removed after intravenous heparin is no longer required.

subcutaneous tissue (Figure 8.5). This will serve as a guide for future dissection in the event that operative closure of the AVF becomes necessary. Most AVFs do not require operative closure as neointimal fibroplasia reduces the volume flow through most and patients remain asymptomatic.

Prior to wound closure, a diligent search for serous accumulation from transected lymphatics is performed. Ligation and coagulation of transected lymphatics are important, especially in the area of dissection around the profunda femoris vein. A closed suction drain is placed in the wound to evacuate any serosanguineous fluid that may accumulate postoperatively. The drain exits through a separate puncture site adjacent to the incision. The wound is closed with running absorbable sutures closing the multiple layers to achieve hemostatic and lymphostatic wound closure and ensure elimination of all dead space.

In patients with operative exposure of the posterior tibial vein, the distal posterior tibial vein is ligated prior to wound closure. A small infusion catheter (such as a pediatric feeding tube) is brought into the wound via a separate stab incision in the skin, and the catheter is inserted and fixed into the proximal posterior tibial vein (Figure 8.5). This catheter is used for postoperative anticoagulation with UFH. A predischarge

phlebogram is generally performed prior to its removal. Postoperative anticoagulation via this catheter ensures maximum concentration of heparin in the thrombectomized veins where it is needed most. A 2-0 monofilament suture is looped around the posterior tibial vein (and catheter) and both ends exit the skin. The ends of the suture are passed through the holes of a sterile button, which is secured snugly to the skin when the catheter is removed. This maneuver obliterates the open end of the proximal posterior tibial vein at the time of catheter removal and eliminates the risk of bleeding. A completion phlebogram is performed to confirm that unobstructed venous drainage is restored to the vena cava.

Antibiotic ointment is applied to all wounds beneath sterile dressings. The patient's leg is wrapped snugly with sterile gauze and multilayered elastic bandages from the base of the toes to the groin. The posterior tibial vein catheter exits between the layers of the bandage. The heparin infusion connected to the catheter is mounted on an IV pole with wheels so that the patient may freely ambulate postoperatively. When the patient is therapeutically anticoagulated on vitamin K antagonists (VKAs), a predischarge phlebogram is performed through the catheter prior to its removal.

Postoperative care

Therapeutic anticoagulation is continued with UFH through the posterior tibial vein catheter. Before removal of the posterior tibial vein catheter, an ascending phlebogram is performed. Oral anticoagulation is begun when the patient awakens and resumes oral intake. Heparin infusion is continued for an overlap of 4 to 5 days and the international normalized ratio (INR) reaches 2 to 3. Oral anticoagulation is continued for a minimum of 1 year.

Intermittent pneumatic compression (IPC) garments are used on both legs postoperatively when the patient is not ambulating. Before discharge, the patient is fitted for 30 to 40 mmHg ankle-gradient below-knee compression stockings and instructed to wear the stockings from the time of awakening in the morning until bedtime at night. Randomized trials have demonstrated a 50% to 55% reduction in postthrombotic morbidity with the use of 30 to 40 mmHg ankle-gradient compression stockings.[31,32]

When the patient is fully recovered and back to baseline activity, a repeat venous duplex and venous function studies are performed to evaluate patency and vein valve function, which serve as baseline studies for future patient evaluation.

The long-term benefits of venous thrombectomy relate to its ability to achieve proximal patency and maintain distal venous valve function. Both are influenced by initial technical success and the avoidance of recurrent thrombosis. Initial success at achieving patency is influenced by timely intervention and attention to technical detail. Pooled data from a number of contemporary reports[16,33–44] of iliofemoral venous thrombectomy indicate that the early and long-term patency rates of the iliofemoral venous segment are 75% to 80% compared to 30% in patients treated with anticoagulation alone[6] (Table 8.3). Femoropopliteal venous valve function is preserved in the majority of patients. Operative series that report femoropopliteal valve competence[16,34,36,40,41,45,46] are summarized in Table 8.3.

Thrombolytic therapy: Systemic

Initial attempts at pharmacologic resolution of acute DVT used systemic thrombolysis. Early studies involving systemic delivery of plasminogen activators resulted in high rates of bleeding complications and less than optimal lytic results. Many patients with infrainguinal DVT were included; therefore, in these trials of systemic thrombolysis, even when lytic therapy was successful, the benefits were not as apparent as those expected following successful treatment of iliofemoral venous thrombosis.

Thirteen studies that compared anticoagulant therapy with systemic thrombolytic therapy for acute DVT have been reported.[33] Patients were evaluated phlebographically both before and after treatment. A pooled analysis of the outcomes showed that only 4% of those treated with anticoagulation alone had significant or complete lysis and 14% had partial lysis (Table 8.4). The remaining 82% had no objective improvement or worsened. Therefore, few patients treated by anticoagulation alone had sufficient early clearing of their thrombus to expect return of vein patency and normal valve function. Forty-five percent of the patients treated with thrombolytic agents had significant or complete clot resolution, and another 18% had partial clearing. Thirty-seven percent failed to improve or worsened. Although lytic therapy had better phlebographic outcomes than anticoagulation alone, the net result is that less than half of the lytic therapy patients had a good or excellent phlebographic result.

Table 8.3 Long-term results of venous thrombectomy with arteriovenous fistula: Iliac vein patency and femoral-popliteal valve competence

No. reports	References	Patients	Follow-up (months)	Iliac vein patency	Femoral-popliteal valve competence
13	16, 33–44	756	55 (mean)	80%	—
7	16, 34, 36, 40, 41, 45, 46	352	45 (mean)	—	63%

Table 8.4 Phlebographic results of anticoagulation versus systemic lytic therapy for acute DVT (13 studies)

Treatment (no.)	Lysis outcome		
	None/worse	Partial	Significant/complete
Heparin (212)	81%	14%	5%
Lytic Rx (253)	40%	15%	45%

Source: Comerota AJ, Gravett MH, J Vasc Surg 2007; 46:1065–1076.
Note: DVT, deep venous thrombosis.

Two of these randomized treatment trials followed patients over the long term. They both found that the majority of patients who were free of postthrombotic symptoms were treated with lytic therapy, whereas the majority of patients with severe postthrombotic morbidity were treated with anticoagulation alone.[48,49] Jeffery et al.[50] found that the patients who were successfully treated with lytic therapy had significant long-term benefit as a result of patent veins with functional valves.

Intrathrombus catheter-directed thrombolysis

There is a physiologic mechanistic reason why direct intrathrombus delivery of plasminogen activators is more successful than systemic thrombolytic therapy. During thrombosis, Glu-plasminogen binds to fibrin, which is then converted to Lys-plasminogen. This molecular modification produces an increased number of binding sites for plasminogen activators, and therefore more efficient production of plasmin following contact with Lys-plasminogen. The basic mechanism of thrombolysis is the activation of fibrin-bound plasminogen with the resultant production of plasmin.[51] It is logical that delivery of the plasminogen activator within the thrombus would be more effective and potentially safer than the systemic infusion of plasminogen activators. Additionally, intrathrombus delivery protects plasminogen activators from circulating inhibitors and, more importantly, protects the active enzyme plasmin from neutralization by circulating antiplasmins. If lysis is accelerated, the overall dose of plasminogen activator and duration of infusion will be reduced, thereby decreasing the risk of treatment-related complications. An important evolution of catheter-directed thrombolysis is the reduction in hourly dose of plasminogen activator and the increase in the volume of solution infused. Efficacy of lysis is dependent upon contact—not concentration—of the plasminogen activator with fibrin-bound plasminogen. Therefore, the greater the volume of solution infused, the more likely the plasminogen activator will contact and bind to plasminogen.

Table 8.5[27,52–69] summarizes reports of catheter-directed thrombolysis for acute DVT. Included in this table are pharmacomechanical techniques used as adjuncts to catheter-directed lytic infusions. Currently, success rates in the range of 80 to 95% can be anticipated. The reported rate of bleeding complications ranges from 5 to 11%. However, distant bleeding is uncommon and intracranial bleeding is a rarity. Most bleeding complications are localized to the venous access site, and recent reports indicate that meaningful bleeding has been reduced to approximately 5% of patients treated. Symptomatic PE during infusion is uncommon and fatal PE a rarity.

The benefit of high-pressure pulse-spray infusion into the thrombus was reported by Chang et al.[70] in a small group of patients with extensive proximal DVT. They used this technique to infuse 50 mg of rt-PA per treatment episode. Following the pulse-spray infusion, patients were returned to their hospital rooms and brought back the following day for repeat phlebographic evaluation and additional treatment if required. Significant or complete lysis was achieved in 11 of 12 extremities, with the remaining patient having 50% to 70% lysis.

National venous registry

The National Venous Registry[56] focused attention of catheter-directed thrombolysis on patients with iliofemoral DVT and formed the basis for

Table 8.5 Review of studies of catheter-directed thrombolysis for acute DVT

Author, year	Total no. of patients (limbs)	Intervention	Significant/ complete resolution (%)	Partial resolution (%)	No resolution (%)	Minor (%)	Major (%)	PE	Death due to Rx (%)
			Results			Complications			
						Bleeding			
Semba et al., 1994[52]	21 (27)	CDT with UK, angioplasty/stenting for residual stenosis	18 (72)	5 (25)	2 (8)	1 (4)	0 (0)	None	None
Semba et al., 1996[53]	32 (41)	CDT with UK, angioplasty/stenting for residual stenosis	21 (32)	9 (28)	2 (6)	0 (0)	0 (0)	None	None
Verhaeghe et al., 1997[54]	24	CDT with rt-PA, stenting for residual stenosis	19 (79)	5 (21)	0 (0)	0 (0)	6 (25)	None	None
Bjarnason et al., 1997[55]	77 (87)	CDT with UK, angioplasty, stenting, thrombectomy, bypass for residual stenosis	69 (793)	0 (0)	18 (21)	11 (14)	5 (6)	1	None
Mewissen et al., 1999[56]	287 (312)	CDT with UK, stenting for residual stenosis; systemic lysis (n = 6)	96 (31)	162 (52)	54 (17)	15 (28)	54 (11)	6	2 (<1)
Comerota et al., 2000[57]	54	CDT with UK or rt-PA, thrombectomy for residual stenosis	14 (26)	28 (52)	6 (11)	8 (15)	4 (7)	1	None
Horne et al., 2000[58]	10	CDT with rt-PA	9 (90)	1 (10)	0 (0)	3 (30)	None	2 (20)	None
Kasirajan et al., 2001[59]	9	CDT with UK, rt-PA, or rPA	7 (78)	1 (11)	1 (11)	NA	NA	NA	NA
AbuRahma et al., 2001[60]	51	CDT with UK or rt-PA, stents/18 Hep/33	15 (83) / 1 (3)	NR / NR	NR / NR	3 (17) / 3 (9)	2 (11) / 2 (6)	None / 2 (6)	None / None
Vedantham et al., 2002[61]	20 (28)	CDT with UK, rt-PA, or rPA, thrombectomy, stenting	23 (82)	NR	NR	None	3 (14)	None	None

(Continued)

Table 8.5 (Continued) Review of studies of catheter-directed thrombolysis for acute DVT

Author, year	Total no. of patients (limbs)	Intervention	Results			Complications			
			Significant/complete resolution (%)	Partial resolution (%)	No resolution (%)	Bleeding		PE	Death due to Rx (%)
						Minor (%)	Major (%)		
Elsharawy et al., 2002[27]	35	CDT with SK, angioplasty, stent/18	13 (72)	5 (28)	0 (0)	None	None	None	None
		Hep/17	2 (12)	8 (47)	7 (41)	None	None	None	None
Castaneda et al., 2002[62]	15	CDT with rPA	15 (100)	NR	NR	None	None	None	None
Grunwald et al., 2004[63]	74 (82)	CDT with UK, tPA, or rPA, angioplasty, stenting	54 (73)	26 (32)	NR	6 (8)	4 (5)	None	None
Laiho et al., 2004[64]	32	CDT with rt-PA/16	8 (50)	5 (31)	NR	4 (25)	2 (13)	2 (13)	None
		Systemic lysis with rt-PA/16	5 (31)	8 (50)	NR	6 (38)	1 (6)	5 (31)	None
Sillesen et al., 2005[65]	45	CDT with rt-PA, angioplasty, stenting	42 (93)	NR	NR	4 (8)	None	1 (2)	None
Jackson et al., 2005[66]	28	CDT with UK or rPA, stenting	5 (18)	20 (72)	NR	2 (7)	None	None	None
Ogawa et al., 2005[67]	24	CDT with UK/10	0 (0)	10 (100)	None	None	None	None	None
		CDT with UK + IPC/14	5 (36)	9 (64)	None	None	None	None	None
Kim et al., 2006[68]	37 (45)	CDT with UK/23	21 (81)	3 (11)	2 (8)	1 (4)	2 (7)	1 (4)	None
		CDT + PMT/14	16 (84)	3 (16)	None	None	1 (5)	1 (5)	None
Lin et al., 2006[69]	93 (98)	CDT with rPA, rt-PA, or UK, angioplasty, stenting/46	32 (70)	14 (30)	5 (11)	2 (4)	1 (2)	None	None
		PMT with rPA, rt-PA, or UK, angioplasty, stenting/52	39 (75)	13 (25)	4 (8)	2 (4)	None	None	None

Note: CDT, catheter-directed thrombolysis; Hep, heparin; IPC, intermittent pneumatic compression; PMT, pharmacomechanical thrombolysis; rPA, recombinant plasminogen activator; rt-PA, recombinant tissue plasminogen activator; tPA, tissue plasminogen activator; UK, urokinase.

many institutions to begin programs of patient management for those presenting with ilio-femoral DVT. While catheter-based techniques have advanced considerably since this report, it remains the largest report of patients treated with lytic therapy for acute DVT, and many of the observations from this study remain valid today. Seventy-one percent of patients treated in the registry had iliofemoral DVT and 25% had femoropopliteal DVT. Intrathrombus catheter-directed infusion of urokinase was the preferred treatment. In the group of patients with acute first-time iliofemoral DVT, 65% had complete clot resolution.

There was a significant correlation ($p < .001$) of thrombus-free survival with the results of initial therapy. At 1 year, 78% of the patients who had complete clot resolution had patent veins versus only 37% of patients who had <50% lysis. This is the first report that suggests a correlation of long-term outcome with initial lytic success of catheter-directed thrombolysis. In the group of patients with first-time iliofemoral DVT who had success-ful thrombolysis, 95% of the veins were patent at 1 year. Initial lytic success also correlated with valve function after 6 months. Thirty-eight percent of patients with <50% thrombolysis had functional venous valves, whereas 72% with complete lysis had normal valve function at 6 months ($p < .02$).

A cohort-controlled quality of life (QOL) study was performed to determine whether lytic therapy altered QOL in patients with iliofemoral DVT.[9] Patients from the same institutions as the National Venous Registry who had iliofemoral DVT treated with anticoagulation as a result of physician pref-erence were compared to those who underwent catheter-directed thrombolysis. All patients who were treated with anticoagulation were candidates for lytic therapy; however, treatment was deter-mined by physician preference. Patients were eval-uated with a validated QOL questionnaire,[71] which was used to query patients at 16 and 22 months after treatment. Ninety-eight patients were evaluated; 68 were treated with catheter-directed thrombolysis and 30 with anticoagulation alone. The results demonstrated that catheter-directed thrombolysis was associated with significantly better QOL than anticoagulation alone. QOL was directly related to initial success of thrombolysis. Patients who had a successful lytic outcome reported a better Health Utilities Index, improved physical function, less stigma of chronic venous disease, less health dis-tress, and fewer overall postthrombotic symptoms. Not surprisingly, those in whom catheter-directed thrombolysis failed had outcomes similar to those of patients treated with anticoagulation alone. A small randomized trial performed by Elsharawy et al.[27] compared catheter-directed thrombo-lysis with anticoagulation alone. Catheter-infused lysis resulted in considerably better outcomes at 6 months with improved patency and vein valve function.

Enden et al.[72] published the results of the CaVenT study, which was an investigator-initiated randomized controlled trial of additional catheter-directed thrombolysis versus anticoagulation alone in patients with a first-time iliofemoral DVT (Table 8.6). Patients were eligible if they presented within 21 days of symptom onset. The primary end-point of this study was postthrombotic syndrome determined by the Villalta score at 24 months and iliofemoral patency at 6 months.

Catheter-directed thrombolysis was performed with the UniFuse catheter (AngioDynamics, Latham, New York). Alteplase was infused at a dose of 0.01 mg/kg/hour for a maximum of 96 hours. The alteplase was prepared by mixing 20 mg in 500 cc of 0.9% NaCl. This would result in a 70 kg man being infused with 0.7 mg of rt-PA in 17.5 cc of infusate. This appears to be an unusually small volume of infusate, which might potentially disad-vantage patients.

Table 8.6 Outcomes of CaVenT study

Endpoint	Additional CDT (N = 90)	Anticoagulation alone (N = 99)	p Value
Iliofemoral patency at 6 months	58 (66%)	45 (47%)	0.012
PTS at 24 months	37 (41%)	55 (56%)	0.047

Source: Data from Enden T, et al., *Lancet* 2012; 379:31–38.

The mean duration of thrombolysis was 24 days. Forty-three percent had complete thrombolysis, 37% had partial, and 10% were deemed unsuccessful. Three percent of patients receiving catheter-directed thrombolysis had major bleeding complications versus none who were randomized to anticoagulation alone. There was an absolute risk reduction in postthrombotic syndrome of 14.4% in patients receiving catheter-directed thrombolysis. Iliofemoral patency at 6 months was achieved in 66% of patients receiving catheter-directed thrombolysis versus 47% receiving anticoagulation alone ($p = .012$). Postthrombotic syndrome was significantly reduced in those randomized to catheter-directed thrombolysis, where it occurred in 41% versus 56% in patients randomized to anticoagulation alone ($p = .047$).

These results demonstrated a significant benefit in those patients receiving additional catheter-directed thrombolysis. The actual benefit would likely have been substantially greater if patients entered into this trial truly had iliofemoral DVT. In reality, only 45% of the patients randomized to catheter-directed thrombolysis and 36% in the anticoagulation alone group had iliofemoral DVT. Therefore, although approximately 60% of patients randomized in this trial had less than iliofemoral DVT, significant benefit was observed. This author believes that the reduction of postthrombotic morbidity would have been substantially greater if indeed all patients in CaVenT had iliofemoral DVT.

A National Institutes of Health (NIH)-sponsored trial, the ATTRACT study,[73] is underway with over 375 patients randomized. It is anticipated that ATTRACT will offer definitive data regarding the benefit of a strategy of catheter-based thrombus removal versus anticoagulation alone for proximal DVT. Patients with acute proximal DVT are stratified according to the distribution of their DVT (iliofemoral or femoropopliteal) and then randomized to a strategy of catheter-based thrombus removal or anticoagulation alone (Figure 8.6). Pharmacomechanical techniques will also be evaluated versus catheter-directed thrombolysis with drip infusion alone.

Available data to date present a compelling argument for catheter-directed thrombolysis. Institutions participating in randomized trials should make every effort to enroll patients who are eligible. Those not participating in trials should adopt a strategy of thrombus removal that **is** based upon evidence available to date.

Patient evaluation

Patients with iliofemoral DVT have a greater stimulus to thrombosis than the majority of patients with DVT, and therefore warrant a search for an underlying etiology. Asymptomatic pulmonary emboli are present in at least 50% of patients. It is important that the PE be recognized early, for up to 25% of asymptomatic pulmonary emboli will subsequently become symptomatic, manifesting as pleuritic chest discomfort once the inflammatory

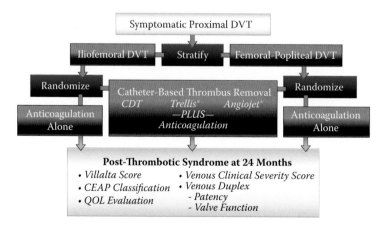

Figure 8.6 Algorithm illustrates the stratification and treatment protocol for acute iliofemoral and femoropopliteal DVT in the ATTRACT study.

pulmonary infarct reaches the parietal surface of the lung. If the PE is not recognized, clinicians often mistakenly assume that the pleuritic symptoms are due to a new PE, and therefore conclude that the patient has failed treatment. A spiral CT scan of the chest with contrast evaluates the pulmonary vasculature for PE and other thoracic pathology (Figure 8.7). The CT scan is extended to the abdomen and pelvis to identify the proximal extent of thrombus and to evaluate for abdominal or pelvic pathology (Figure 8.8). We also perform a rapid CT scan of the brain to assess for intracranial pathology. The CT scan has been an important addition to the evaluation of these patients, as we have found serious unsuspected pathology with surprising frequency. Renal cell carcinoma, adrenal tumors, retroperitoneal lymphoma, hepatic metastases, iliac vein aneurysms, and vena caval atresia have all been identified. An evaluation for an underlying thrombophilia is not performed, as it will rarely change patient care. However, in patients with an unprovoked DVT, a thrombophilia evaluation of first-degree female relatives of childbearing potential is recommended.

Technique

The preferred approach in most patients with iliofemoral DVT is through an ultrasound-guided popliteal vein puncture with antegrade passage of the infusion catheter. Through this approach, physicians can incorporate adjunctive mechanical thrombectomy techniques.

If the popliteal vein is thrombosed, an additional catheter is placed through an ultrasound-guided tibial vein puncture. Using catheters that achieve long segments of thrombus infusion is advised. This author believes it is valuable to restore venous drainage into the popliteal vein if infrapopliteal thrombosis exists.

Frequently patients with iliofemoral DVT have such high venous pressures that pressure on the ultrasound probe fails to compress the distal femoral, popliteal, and calf veins. A falsely positive diagnosis of venous thrombosis is made, which is not recognized until a phlebogram is performed once the vein is entered.

As mentioned before, lower doses of plasminogen activator are used, dissolving 1 mg of rt-PA into 50 to 100 mL of saline. Up to 100 cc per hour are infused. The larger volume is intended to saturate the thrombus, thereby contacting more

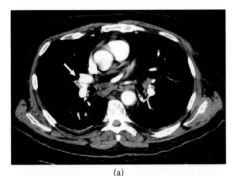

(a)

(b)

Figure 8.7 Contrast-enhanced CT of the chest often reveals unsuspected pathology, including (a) an asymptomatic PE (arrow) and (b) mediastinal lymph nodes. Note posterior tracheal compression by enlarged lymph nodes.

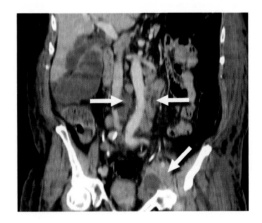

Figure 8.8 Extending the CT to the abdomen and pelvis not only identifies the proximal extent of thrombus but evaluates for abdominal or pelvic pathology, as was the case in this patient with previously undiagnosed retroperitoneal and pelvic lymphadenopathy (arrows).

plasminogen activator to the fibrin-bound plasminogen. Phlebograms are obtained at 12-hour intervals and are used to monitor the success of lysis and reposition the catheters if necessary. Vena caval filters are not routinely used but are recommended for patients with free-floating thrombus in the vena cava. A retrievable filter can be used in patients in whom only temporary protection is needed.

Following successful thrombolysis, the venous system is examined with completion phlebography. If a stenosis exists, which is frequently observed in the common iliac vein where it is compressed by the right common iliac artery, the vein is dilated and stented if necessary. The addition of intravascular ultrasonography has improved the evaluation of iliac compression and the precision of stent placement when these lesions are corrected. Residual areas of stenosis must be corrected for long-term success; otherwise, the patient faces a high risk of rethrombosis. If a stent is used, it should be sized appropriate to the normal diameter of the common iliac vein.

Pharmacomechanical thrombolysis

Although good results are achieved with catheter-directed drip thrombolysis, treatment times are often unacceptably long, and therefore bleeding risk and cost associated with therapy are high. This was succinctly characterized by Sillesen and colleagues[74] when they reported that 93% of their patients were successfully treated with the drip technique and discharged with patent veins, and that >90% of the patients discharged with patent veins had normal venous valve function. The patients treated in this series had relatively acute thrombus, as the mean duration of symptoms was just 7 days. Patients with symptoms exceeding 14 days were excluded. Therefore, lysis would be expected to occur quickly in these patients. However, treatment times for catheter-directed thrombolysis averaged 71 hours, despite the short duration of symptoms. Prolonged treatment times are logistically difficult for many practitioners and medical centers. The associated cost is high because patients receiving lytic therapy are usually monitored in intensive care units. Therefore, it is natural that percutaneous mechanical techniques

and methods that combine mechanical and pharmacologic (lytic) therapy have been developed in an effort to reduce treatment times, reduce complications, and improve outcomes.

Endovascular mechanical thrombectomy

The purpose of mechanical techniques, either alone or in combination with catheter-directed infusion, is to more rapidly clear thrombus from the venous system. Vedantham et al.[61] evaluated the effectiveness of mechanical thrombectomy alone or in combination with pharmacomechanical thrombolysis in 28 limbs of patients with acute DVT. They evaluated multiple devices, including the Amplatz (ev3, Plymouth, Minnesota), AngioJet (Medrad, Minneapolis, Minnesota), Trerotola (Arrow International, Reading, Pennsylvania), and Oasis (Boston Scientific/Medi-tek, Natick, Massachusetts) catheters. Venographic scoring was performed at each step of the procedure. Twenty-six percent of the thrombus was removed by mechanical thrombectomy alone, whereas adding a plasminogen activator to the infusion solution improved thrombus removal to 82%. This analysis includes patients with chronic occlusion who did not respond at all; therefore, one would expect better results in patients with only acute thrombus. Mechanical thrombectomy alone was highly successful in removing thrombus that develops during the procedure, which is generally gelatinous and not cross-linked with factor XIIIa. The average infusion time was approximately

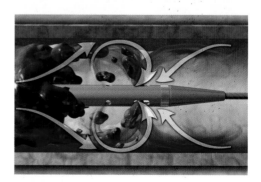

Figure 8.9 The AngioJet rheolytic thrombectomy catheter.

17 hours per limb and 14% of patients had minor bleeding complications.

Lin et al.[69] reported their 8-year experience with pharmacomechanical thrombolysis via a rheolytic thrombectomy catheter (Figure 8.9). Of their 98 patients, 46 received thrombolysis alone and 52 underwent pharmacomechanical thrombolysis. Pharmacomechanical lysis with the AngioJet catheter was associated with significantly fewer phlebograms, shorter intensive care unit stays, shorter hospital stays, and fewer blood transfusions. Bleeding complications were not different between the two groups.

Kasirajan et al.[59] evaluated a smaller group of patients treated by rheolytic thrombectomy. They demonstrated that the rheolytic catheter using saline alone was less effective than when a plasminogen activator–saline solution was used.

Ultrasound-accelerated thrombolysis

Parikh et al.[76] reported the initial registry experience with ultrasound-accelerated thrombolysis in 53 patients treated for acute DVT with the EKOS catheter (EKOS Corp, Bothell, Washington) (Figure 8.10). Both upper- and lower-extremity DVT patients were included, which causes problems in evaluating efficacy for lower-extremity DVT. Additionally, a variety of lytic agents were used. Complete lysis (≥90%) was observed in 70% of patients and overall lysis (complete and partial) in 91%. The median infusion time was 22 hours, and 4% of the patients had major complications, which were essentially puncture site hematomas. The authors' impression was that when compared

with historical controls, treatment time and dose of lytic agents were reduced with ultrasound-accelerated thrombolysis.

However, Baker et al.[77] reported a single-center retrospective analysis of CDT ($N = 19$) versus ultrasound-accelerated thrombolysis ($N = 64$) in patients with iliofemoral DVT. The baseline parameters, extent of DVT, and time since onset of symptoms did not differ between groups. Both treatment groups had a similar and substantial resolution of thrombus load (CDT = 89%, ultrasound = 82%; $p = .560$). There were no significant differences in the lytic drug infusion rate, dose of plasminogen activator, infusion time, or use of adjunctive procedures between groups. Major and minor bleeding complications were observed in 8.4 and 4.8% of patients and were not different between groups. A properly designed randomized trial is needed to properly evaluate this potentially important therapeutic option.

Isolated segmental pharmacomechanical thrombolysis

The technique of segmenting the section of thrombosed venous system to be treated with catheter-directed pharmacomechanical techniques can be achieved with the Trellis catheter (Covidien, Santa Clara, California) (Figure 8.11). This double-balloon catheter is inserted into the thrombosed venous segment with the proximal balloon positioned at the upper edge (cephalic end) of the thrombus. When the balloons are inflated,

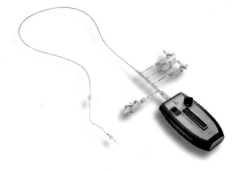

Figure 8.11 The Trellis isolated, segmental pharmacomechanical thrombolysis catheter. (Courtesy of Covidien.)

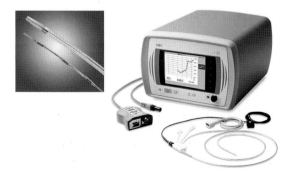

Figure 8.10 EKOS catheter. (Courtesy of EKOS Corp.)

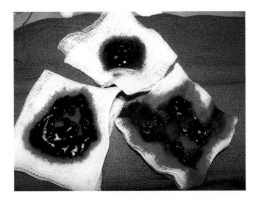

Figure 8.12 Liquefied, fragmented thrombus aspirated through the sheath after isolated, segmental pharmacomechanical thrombolysis.

a plasminogen activator is infused into the thrombosed segment isolated by the two balloons. The intervening catheter assumes a spiral configuration and spins at approximately 3500 rpm for 15 to 20 minutes. The liquefied and fragmented thrombus can be aspirated via the infusion sheath (Figure 8.12) and treatment success evaluated by repeat segmental phlebography. If successful, the catheter is repositioned and additional thrombosed segments are treated. If residual thrombus persists, repeat treatment or other appropriate intervention (rheolytic thrombectomy, ultrasound-accelerated thrombolysis, balloon angioplasty/stenting) is performed.

Martinez et al.[78] reviewed 52 consecutive limbs treated for iliofemoral DVT, the first 27 with catheter-directed thrombolysis and the following 25 with isolated segmental pharmacomechanical thrombolysis (ISPMT) plus catheter-directed thrombolysis when necessary. Thrombus burden and treatment outcomes were quantified. Ninety-three percent of the patients were treated with rt-PA, and venoplasty and stenting were used to correct underlying stenoses. All patients received long-term therapeutic anticoagulation. Sixteen of the 27 legs treated by catheter-directed thrombolysis required other adjunctive mechanical techniques to clear the thrombus, such as the AngioJet, ultrasound-accelerated lysis, or pulse-spray techniques, whereas only 7 of the 25 limbs treated with ISPMT required additional adjunctive techniques. A larger percentage of the thrombus was removed with ISPMT than with catheter-directed thrombolysis. Complete lysis (≥90%) was achieved in 11%

of the limbs in the catheter-directed lysis group, as opposed to 28% of the limbs treated with ISPMT ($p = .077$). Treatment time was shorter ($p < .001$) and the rt-PA dose was lower ($p = .009$) with ISPMT. Hospital and intensive care unit lengths of stay were no different, which appeared to be the result of underlying patient comorbid conditions. Using the Trellis catheter only, success was achieved in a single setting in 18%, which is consistent with the observations of O'Sullivan and associates.[79] Bleeding complications occurred in 5% of patients undergoing catheter-directed thrombolysis alone and 5% of patients treated by ISPMT.

Our current approach is to use ISPMT to eliminate as much thrombus as possible as early as possible. If segmented thrombus remains, rheolytic thrombectomy with the AngioJet is helpful. If patients require extended infusion of the plasminogen activator, my preference is to deliver that infusion via the ultrasound-accelerated thrombolysis system (EKOS Lysus system) (Figure 8.13a–k).

Recurrent DVT

Recurrent DVT is a particularly morbid condition that exposes the patient to a substantially higher risk of postthrombotic syndrome and obligates the patient to indefinite anticoagulation.

Douketis et al.[80] followed 1149 consecutive patients with lower-extremity DVT. They reported that patients with iliofemoral DVT had a significantly higher recurrence rate than patients with infrainguinal DVT. In their series, 12% of patients had recurrent DVT within 3 months. This is a particularly troublesome observation since the recurrence occurred while patients were being treated with anticoagulation.

In general, it is expected that 30 to 40% of patients will develop a recurrent DVT within 5 to 10 years of their initial event. It is instructive to observe that in Baekgaard et al.'s prospective evaluation of 103 patients treated for iliofemoral DVT with catheter-directed thrombolysis, only 6% developed recurrence during follow-up.[81] Aziz et al.[82] reviewed 75 consecutive patients with iliofemoral DVT who were treated with catheter-directed thrombolysis. These patients were followed for a mean of 35 months. Recurrent DVT

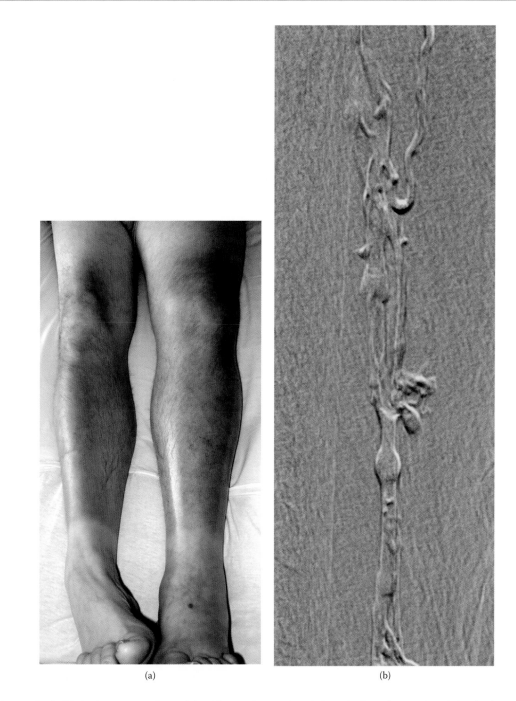

(a) (b)

Figure 8.13 (a) Patient presenting with phlegmasia cerulea dolens 1 day after major abdominal surgery. Ascending phlebogram shows extensive venous thrombosis confirming the venous ultrasound findings of clot extending from the (b) calf veins.

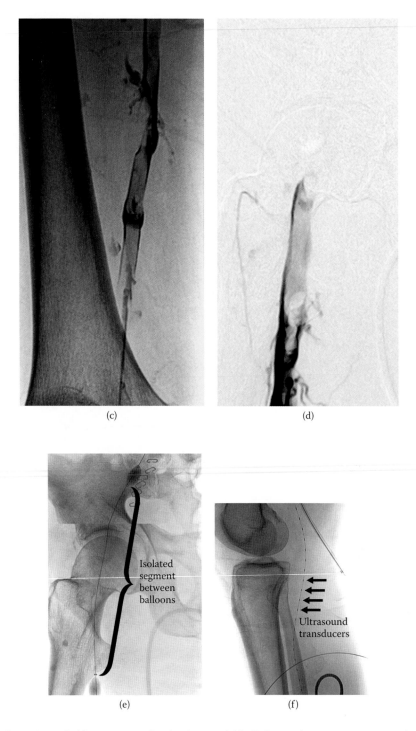

Figure 8.13 (Continued) (c) Femoropopliteal veins, and (d) iliofemoral venous segment. The patient was treated with isolated, segmental pharmacomechanical thrombolysis using the (e) Trellis catheter and overnight infusion with (f) ultrasound-accelerated thrombolysis using the EKOS Lysus catheter. Residual segmented thrombus was cleared with the rheolytic AngioJet catheter.

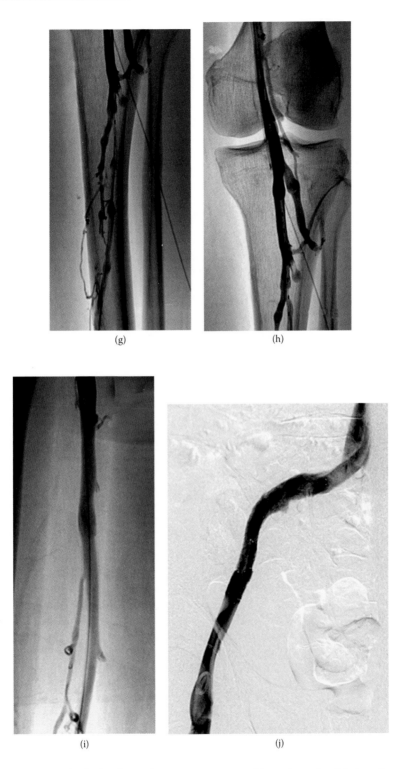

(g)

(h)

(i)

(j)

Figure 8.13 (*Continued*) (g–j) The iliac veins were compressed by enlarged pelvic lymph nodes and were stented. A completion phlebogram shows patent veins from the calf to the vena cava. The patient was diagnosed with lymphoma and received chemotherapy with good success.

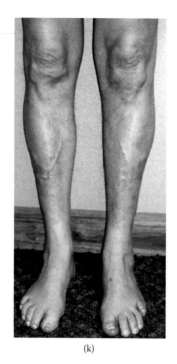

(k)

Figure 8.13 (*Continued*) (k) At 16 months, the patient was asymptomatic and had a patent venous system with functional valves.

occurred in 9% of patients. However, when patients were broken into treatment groups, namely, <50% of residual thrombus or ≥50% of residual thrombus at the completion of treatment, the recurrence rates between these groups were significantly different. The mean amount of residual thrombus in the <50% group was 18% versus 60% in the ≥50% group. Patients with substantial lysis had a 5% recurrence rate, whereas those who had the majority of thrombus remaining after catheter-directed thrombolysis experienced a 50% recurrent DVT rate ($p = .0014$).

These observational data strongly suggest that clearing the thrombus not only restores patency and reduces postthrombotic morbidity but also reduces the risk of recurrent DVT.

REFERENCES

1. Qvarfordt P, Eklof B, Ohlin P. Intramuscular pressure in the lower leg in deep vein thrombosis and phlegmasia cerulae dolens. *Ann Surg* 1983; 197:450–453.

2. Labropoulos N, Volteas N, Leon M, et al. The role of venous outflow obstruction in patients with chronic venous dysfunction. *Arch Surg* 1997; 132:46–51.

3. Kearon C, Kahn SR, Agnelli G, Goldhaber SZ, Raskob G, Comerota AJ. Antithrombotic therapy for venous thromboembolic disease: ACCP evidence-based clinical practice guidelines (8th ed). *Chest* 2008; 133:454S–545S.

4. Jaff MR, McMurtry MS, Archer SL, et al. Management of massive and submassive pulmonary embolism, iliofemoral deep vein thrombosis, and chronic thromboembolic pulmonary hypertension: a scientific statement from the American Heart Association. *Circulation* 2011; 123:1788–1830.

5. Goldhaber SZ, Buring JE, Lipnick RJ, Hennekens CH. Pooled analyses of randomized trials of streptokinase and heparin in phlebographically documented acute deep venous thrombosis. *Am J Med* 1984; 76:393–397.

6. O'Donnell TF, Browse NL, Burnand KG, Thomas ML. The socioeconomic effects of an iliofemoral venous thrombosis. *J Surg Res* 1977; 22:483–488.

7. Akesson H, Brudin L, Dahlstrom JA, Eklof B, Ohlin P, Plate G. Venous function assessed during a 5 year period after acute ilio-femoral venous thrombosis treated with anticoagulation. *Eur J Vasc Surg* 1990; 4:43–48.

8. Delis KT, Bountouroglou D, Mansfield AO. Venous claudication in iliofemoral thrombosis: long-term effects on venous hemodynamics, clinical status, and quality of life. *Ann Surg* 2004; 239:118–126.

9. Comerota AJ, Throm RC, Mathias SD, Haughton S, Mewissen M. Catheter-directed thrombolysis for iliofemoral deep venous thrombosis improves health-related quality of life. *J Vasc Surg* 2000; 32:130–137.

10. Cho JS, Martelli E, Mozes G, Miller VM, Gloviczki P. Effects of thrombolysis and venous thrombectomy on valvular competence, thrombogenicity, venous wall morphology, and function. *J Vasc Surg* 1998; 28:787–799.

11. Rhodes JM, Cho JS, Gloviczki P, Mozes G, Rolle R, Miller VM. Thrombolysis for experimental deep venous thrombosis maintains valvular competence and vasoreactivity. *J Vasc Surg* 2000; 31:1193–1205.

12. Meissner MH, Manzo RA, Bergelin RO, Markel A, Strandness DE Jr. Deep venous insufficiency: the relationship between lysis and subsequent reflux. *J Vasc Surg* 1993; 18:596–605.

13. Markel A, Manzo RA, Bergelin RO, Strandness DE Jr. Valvular reflux after deep vein thrombosis: incidence and time of occurrence. *J Vasc Surg* 1992; 15:377–382.

14. Johnson BF, Manzo RA, Bergelin RO, Strandness DE Jr. Relationship between changes in the deep venous system and the development of the postthrombotic syndrome after an acute episode of lower limb deep vein thrombosis: a one- to six-year follow-up. *J Vasc Surg* 1995; 21:307–312.

15. Plate G, Akesson H, Einarsson E, Ohlin P, Eklof B. Long-term results of venous thrombectomy combined with a temporary arterio-venous fistula. *Eur J Vasc Surg* 1990; 4:483–489.

16. Plate G, Einarsson E, Ohlin P, Jensen R, Qvarfordt P, Eklof B. Thrombectomy with temporary arteriovenous fistula: the treatment of choice in acute iliofemoral venous thrombosis. *J Vasc Surg* 1984; 1:867–876.

17. Plate G, Eklof B, Norgren L, Ohlin P, Dahlstrom JA. Venous thrombectomy for iliofemoral vein thrombosis—10-year results of a prospective randomised study. *Eur J Vasc Endovasc Surg* 1997; 14:367–374.

18. Shull KC, Nicolaides AN, Fernandes é Fernandes J, et al. Significance of popliteal reflux in relation to ambulatory venous pressure and ulceration. *Arch Surg* 1979; 114:1304–1306.

19. Nicolaides AN, Schull K, Fernandes E. Ambulatory venous pressure: new information. In Nicolaides AN, Yao JS (eds.), *Investigation of vascular disorders*. New York: Churchill Livingstone, 1981; 488–494.

20. Eklof B, Rutherford RB, Bergan JJ, et al. Revision of the CEAP classification for chronic venous disorders: consensus statement. *J Vasc Surg* 2004; 40:1248–1252.

21. Welkie JF, Comerota AJ, Katz ML, Aldridge SC, Kerr RP, White JV. Hemodynamic deterioration in chronic venous disease. *J Vasc Surg* 1992; 16:733–740.

22. Comerota AJ, Grewal NK, Thakur S, Assi Z. Endovenectomy of the common femoral vein and intraoperative iliac vein recanalization for chronic iliofemoral venous occlusion. *J Vasc Surg* 2010; 52:243–247.

23. Killewich LA, Bedford GR, Beach KW, Strandness DE Jr. Spontaneous lysis of deep venous thrombi: rate and outcome. *J Vasc Surg* 1989; 9:89–97.

24. Sevitt S. The structure and growth of valve-pocket thrombi in femoral veins. *J Clin Pathol* 1974; 27:517–528.

25. Sevitt S. The mechanisms of canalisation in deep vein thrombosis. *J Pathol* 1973; 110:153–165.

26. Brooks EG, Trotman W, Wadsworth MP, et al. Valves of the deep venous system: an overlooked risk factor. *Blood* 2009; 114:1276–1279.

27. Elsharawy M, Elzayat E. Early results of thrombolysis vs anticoagulation in ilio-femoral venous thrombosis. A randomised clinical trial. *Eur J Vasc Endovasc Surg* 2002; 24:209–214.

28. Buller HR, Agnelli G, Hull RD, Hyers TM, Prins MH, Raskob GE. Antithrombotic therapy for venous thromboembolic disease: the Seventh ACCP Conference on Antithrombotic and Thrombolytic Therapy. *Chest* 2004; 126:401S–428S.

29. Comerota AJ, Gale SS. Technique of contemporary iliofemoral and infrainguinal venous thrombectomy. *J Vasc Surg* 2006; 43:185–191.

30. Eklof B, Juhan C. Revival of thrombectomy in the management of acute iliofemoral venous thrombosis. *Contemp Surg* 1992; 40:21.

31. Brandjes DP, Buller HR, Heijboer H, et al. Randomised trial of effect of compression stockings in patients with symptomatic proximal-vein thrombosis. *Lancet* 1997; 349:759–762.

32. Prandoni P, Lensing AW, Prins MH, et al. Below-knee elastic compression stockings to prevent the post-thrombotic syndrome: a randomized, controlled trial. *Ann Intern Med* 2004; 141:249–256.

33. Piquet P. Traitement chirurgical des thromboses iliocaves: exigences et resultats. In Kieffer E (ed.), *Chirurgie de la Veine Cave Inferieure et de Ses Branches*. Paris: Expansion Scientifique Francaise, 1985; 210–216.

34. Einarsson E, Albrechtsson U, Eklof B, Norgren L. Follow-up evaluation of venous morphologic factors and function after thrombectomy and temporary arteriovenous fistula in thrombosis of iliofemoral vein. *Surg Gynecol Obstet* 1986; 163:111–116.

35. Vollmar JF. Robert May memorial lecture: advances in reconstructive venous surgery. *Int Angiol* 1986; 5:117–129.

36. Juhan C, Alimi Y, Di Mauro P, Hartung O. Surgical venous thrombectomy. *Cardiovasc Surg* 1999; 7:586–590.

37. Torngren S, Swedenborg J. Thrombectomy and temporary arterio-venous fistula for ilio-femoral venous thrombosis. *Int Angiol* 1988; 7:14–18.

38. Rasmussen A, Mogensen K, Nissen FH, Wadt J, Skibsted L. Acute iliofemoral venous thrombosis. 26 cases treated with thrombectomy, temporary arteriovenous fistula and anticoagulants. *Ugeskr Laeger* 1990; 152:2928–2930.

39. Eklof B, Kistner RL. Is there a role for thrombectomy in iliofemoral venous thrombosis? *Semin Vasc Surg* 1996; 9:34–45.

40. Neglen P, al-Hassan HK, Endrys J, Nazzal MM, Christenson JT, Eklof B. Iliofemoral venous thrombectomy followed by percutaneous closure of the temporary arteriovenous fistula. *Surgery* 1991; 110:493–499.

41. Meissner AJ, Huszcza S. Surgical strategy for management of deep venous thrombosis of the lower extremities. *World J Surg* 1996; 20:1149–1155.

42. Pillny M, Sandmann W, Luther B, et al. Deep venous thrombosis during pregnancy and after delivery: indications for and results of thrombectomy. *J Vasc Surg* 2003; 37:528–532.

43. Hartung O, Benmiloud F, Barthelemy P, et al. Late results of surgical venous thrombectomy with iliocaval stenting. *J Vasc Surg* 2008; 47:381–7.

44. Holper P, Kotelis D, Attigah N, et al. Long-term results after surgical thrombectomy and simultaneous stenting for symptomatic iliofemoral venous thrombosis. *Eur J Vasc Endovasc Surg* 2010; 39:349–55.

45. Ganger KH, Nachbur BH, Ris HB, Zurbrugg H. Surgical thrombectomy versus conservative treatment for deep venous thrombosis; functional comparison of long-term results. *Eur J Vasc Surg* 1989; 3:529–38.

46 Kniemeyer HW, Sandmann W, Schwindt C, et al. Thrombectomy with arteriovenous fistula for embolizing deep venous thrombosis: an alternative therapy for prevention of recurrent pulmonary embolism. *Clin Investig* 1993; 72:40–5.

47. Comerota AJ, Gravett MH. Iliofemoral venous thrombosis. *J Vasc Surg* 2007; 46:1065–1076.

48. Elliot MS, Immelman EJ, Jeffery P, et al. A comparative randomized trial of heparin versus streptokinase in the treatment of acute proximal venous thrombosis: an interim report of a prospective trial. *Br J Surg* 1979 Dec; 66:838–43.

49. Arnesen H, Hoiseth A, Ly B. Streptokinase of heparin in the treatment of deep vein thrombosis. Follow-up results of a prospective study. *Acta Med Scand* 1982; 211: 65–8.

50. Jeffery P, Immelman EJ, Amoore J. Treatment of deep vein thrombosis with heparin or streptokinase: long-term venous function assessment. In *Proceedings of the Second International Vascular Symposium*, 1989: abstract S20.3.

51. Alkjaersig N, Fletcher AP, Sherry S. The mechanism of clot dissolution by plasmin. *J Clin Invest* 1959; 38:1086–1095.

52. Semba CP, Dake MD. Iliofemoral deep venous thrombosis: aggressive therapy with catheter-directed thrombolysis. *Radiology* 1994 May;191(2):487–94.

53. Semba CP, Dake MD. Catheter-directed thrombolysis for iliofemoral venous thrombosis. *Semin Vasc Surg* 1996 Mar; 9:26–33.

54. Verhaeghe R, Stockx L, Lacroix H, Vermylen J, Baert AL. Catheter-directed lysis of iliofemoral vein thrombosis with use of rt-PA. *Eur Radiol* 1997; 7:996–1001.

55. Bjarnason H, Kruse JR, Asinger DA, et al. Iliofemoral deep venous thrombosis: safety and efficacy outcome during 5 years of catheter-directed thrombolytic therapy. *J Vasc Interv Radiol* 1997 May; 8:405–418.

56. Mewissen MW, Seabrook GR, Meissner MH, et al. Catheter-directed thrombolysis for lower extremity deep venous thrombosis: report of a national multicenter registry. *Radiology* 1999 Apr; 211:39–49.

57. Comerota AJ, Kagan SA. Catheter-directed thrombolysis for the treatment of acute iliofemoral deep venous thrombosis. *Phlebology* 2001; 15:149–155.

58. Horne MK, III, Mayo DJ, Cannon RO, III, et al. Intraclot recombinant tissue plasminogen activator in the treatment of deep venous thrombosis of the lower and upper extremities. *Am J Med* 2000 Feb 15; 108:251–255.

59. Kasirajan K, Gray B, Ouriel K. Percutaneous AngioJet thrombectomy in the management of extensive deep venous thrombosis. *J Vasc Interv Radiol* 2001 Feb; 12:179–185.

60. AbuRahma AF, Perkins SE, Wulu JT, Ng HK. Iliofemoral deep vein thrombosis: conventional therapy versus lysis and percutaneous transluminal angioplasty and stenting. *Ann Surg* 2001 Jun; 233:752–760.

61. Vedantham S, Vesely TM, Parti N, et al. Lower extremity venous thrombolysis with adjunctive mechanical thrombectomy. *J Vasc Interv Radiol* 2002 Oct;13:1001–1008.

62. Castaneda F, Li R, Young K, Swischuk JL, Smouse B, Brady T. Catheter-directed thrombolysis in deep venous thrombosis with use of reteplase: immediate results and complications from a pilot study. *J Vasc Interv Radiol* 2002 Jun; 13:577–580.

63. Grunwald MR, Hofmann LV. Comparison of urokinase, alteplase, and reteplase for catheter-directed thrombolysis of deep venous thrombosis. *J Vasc Interv Radiol* 2004 Apr; 15:347–352.

64. Laiho MK, Oinonen A, Sugano N, et al. Preservation of venous valve function after catheter-directed and systemic thrombolysis for deep venous thrombosis. *Eur J Vasc Endovasc Surg* 2004 Oct; 28:391–396.

65. Sillesen H, Just S, Jorgensen M, Baekgaard N. Catheter-directed thrombolysis for treatment of ilio-femoral deep venous thrombosis is durable, preserves venous valve function and may prevent chronic venous insufficiency. *Eur J Vasc Endovasc Surg* 2005; 30:556–562.

66. Jackson LS, Wang XJ, Dudrick SJ, Gersten GD. Catheter-directed thrombolysis and/or thrombectomy with selective endovascular stenting as alternatives to systemic anticoagulation for treatment of acute deep vein thrombosis. *Am J Surg* 2005 Dec; 190:864–868.

67. Ogawa T, Hoshino S, Midorikawa H, Sato K. Intermittent pneumatic compression of the foot and calf improves the outcome of catheter-directed thrombolysis using low-dose urokinase in patients with acute proximal venous thrombosis of the leg. *J Vasc Surg* 2005 Nov; 42:940–944.

68. Kim HS, Patra A, Paxton BE, Khan J, Streiff MB. Adjunctive percutaneous mechanical thrombectomy for lower-extremity deep vein thrombosis: clinical and economic outcomes. *J Vasc Interv Radiol* 2006 Jul; 17:1099–1104.

69. Lin PH, Zhou W, Dardik A, et al. Catheter-direct thrombolysis versus pharmaco-mechanical thrombectomy for treatment of symptomatic lower extremity deep venous thrombosis. *Am J Surg* 2006 Dec; 192:782–788.

70. Chang R, Cannon RO, III, Chen CC, et al. Daily catheter-directed single dosing of t-PA in treatment of acute deep venous thrombosis of the lower extremity. *J Vasc Interv Radiol* 2001 Feb; 12:247–252.

71. Mathias SD, Prebil LA, Putterman CG, Chmiel JJ, Throm RC, Comerota AJ. A health-related quality of life measure in patients with deep vein thrombosis: a validation study. *Drug Inf J* 1999; 33:1173–1187.

72. Enden T, Haig Y, Klow NE, et al. Long-term outcome after additional catheter-directed thrombolysis versus standard treatment for acute iliofemoral deep vein thrombosis (the CaVenT study): a randomised controlled trial. *Lancet* 2012; 379:31–38.

73. Comerota AJ. The ATTRACT trial: rationale for early intervention for iliofemoral DVT. *Perspect Vasc Surg Endovasc Ther* 2009; 21: 221–224.

74. Sillesen H, Just S, Jorgensen M, Baekgaard N. Catheter-directed thrombolysis for treatment of ilio femoral deep venous thrombosis is durable, preserves venous valve function and may prevent chronic venous insufficiency. *Eur J Vasc Endovasc Surg* 2005; 30:556–562.

75. Parikh S, Motarjeme A, McNamara T, et al. Ultrasound-accelerated thrombolysis for the treatment of deep vein thrombosis: initial clinical experience. *J Vasc Interv Radiol* 2008; 19:521–528.

76. Baker R, Samuels S, Benenati JF, Powell A, Uthoff H. Ultrasound-accelerated vs standard catheter-directed thrombolysis-A comparative study in patients with iliofemoral deep vein thrombosis. *J Vasc Interv Radiol* 2012; 23:1460–1466.

77. Martinez J, Comerota AJ, Kazanjian S, DiSalle RS, Sepanski DM, Assi Z. The quantitative benefit of isolated, segmental, pharmaco-mechanical thrombolysis for iliofemoral DVT. *J Vasc Surg* 2008; 48:1532–1537.

78. O'Sullivan GJ, Lohan DG, Gough N, Cronin CG, Kee ST. Pharmacomechanical thrombectomy of acute deep vein thrombosis with the Trellis-8 isolated thrombolysis catheter. *J Vasc Interv Radiol* 2007; 18:715–724.

79. Douketis JD, Crowther MA, Foster GA, Ginsberg JS. Does the location of thrombosis determine the risk of disease recurrence in patients with proximal deep vein thrombosis? *Am J Med* 2001; 110:515–519.

80. Baekgaard N, Broholm R, Just S, Jorgensen M, Jensen LP. Long-term results using catheterdirected thrombolysis in 103 lower limbs with acute iliofemoral venous thrombosis. *Eur J Vasc Endovasc Surg* 2010; 39:112–117.

81. Aziz F, Comerota AJ. Quantity of residual thrombus after successful catheter-directed thrombolysis for iliofemoral deep venous thrombosis correlates with recurrence. *Eur J Vasc Endovasc Surg* 2012; 44: 210–213.

9

Inferior vena cava filters

Overview

The majority of patients diagnosed with deep vein thrombosis (DVT) or pulmonary embolism (PE) are effectively managed with conventional anticoagulation.[1] However, patients who have a contraindication to anticoagulation or in whom anticoagulation has failed cannot be effectively managed with conventional pharmacotherapy; in these cases, vena caval filtration becomes an option.

The use of inferior vena caval (IVC) filters has increased substantially during the past two decades as a result of advances in technology, which have improved the ease of insertion and overall success rates. Coupling ease of insertion with generous reimbursement, the number of caval filters being inserted for other than recognized indications has increased considerably. Since many referring physicians and many physicians who perform filter insertion do not have an interest in managing the primary venous thromboembolism (VTE), IVC filters are frequently chosen as the preferred management option.

Currently in the United States, 13 filters are approved for use.[2] Although current data are not available, it would be reasonable to think that during the last 20 years, the use of vena caval filters has increased at least by a factor of 8 to 10, possibly more. IVC filters are likely to be the most common implanted device in the United States and probably the world. The true percentage of patients with confirmed venous thromboembolic complications who require caval filters is not known. It has been estimated that filters are placed in as many as 11%

of patients with VTE,[3] and since the introduction of temporary or "optional" filters, numbers are rising. The per-capita number of caval filters placed in the United States is substantially higher (more than 20 times higher) than the number of filters placed in Sweden (or other countries), despite a similar incidence of VTE and comparable per capita VTE fatality rates.

In data obtained from the National Hospital Discharge Survey from 1997 to 1999, 45% of IVC filters were placed in patients with DVT alone, 36% in patients with PE, and 19% in patients without either DVT or PE.[3] Based upon personal observation and discussion with colleagues, this percentage of "prophylactic" filters (filters placed without DVT or PE) is rapidly escalating.

Indications

Indications for vena caval filters can be categorized as (1) absolute, (2) relative, and (3) prophylactic. In reality, all vena caval filters are prophylactic, to prevent future PE. However, this term is used to describe the indication for patients who have no identifiable PE or DVT.

Absolute indications are (1) venous thromboembolic complications associated with a contraindication to anticoagulation, (2) documented failure of anticoagulation, (3) complications of anticoagulation in patients being treated for VTE, and (4) at the time of open pulmonary thromboembolectomy.[4] Evidence suggests that most patients treated with IVC filters have none of the three accepted absolute indications.[4]

Relative indications exist when patients have a venous thromboembolic event and the risk of PE remains high, despite anticoagulation. This includes patients with iliocaval venous thrombosis, a large free-floating thrombus in the vena cava or iliac veins, massive PE, recurrent PE in the presence of a filter, patients with DVT and a limited cardiopulmonary reserve, patients undergoing lysis for iliocaval DVT with vena caval thrombus, patients with DVT who fall, and those suspected to be noncompliant with anticoagulation.[4]

Prophylactic indications exist in patients who do not have DVT or PE, but in whom the perceived risk of a venous thromboembolic complication is high and the efficacy of established methods of prophylaxis is considered poor (those at risk of pelvic vein thrombosis).

Filter types

Until 2003, all vena caval filters were considered permanent. Since then, retrievable (optional) filters have become available. The nonpermanent filters have been called temporary, retrievable, removable, convertible, and optional. The appropriate nomenclature for most of these removable filters is now optional. The term means that these filters offer the option to be removed, if appropriate, or leave permanently, if indicated. The true temporary filter is one that *must* be removed within a given period of time, since it is externally tethered while in place.

The intended use of a vena caval filter has specific implications regarding its design. Filters designed to be removed will not be firmly attached to the wall of the vena cava and may be at increased risk of migration. Conversely, permanent filters are generally more securely attached, and therefore more difficult to remove. Clinicians should be aware of the design modifications and their implications when selecting a filter to use.

Clinical decision making

When optional filters are used, it is assumed that the patient requires only temporary protection and that a permanent filter will be associated with more harm than transient caval filtration. The rationale

for nonpermanent vena caval filters is that the benefit of removal outweighs the harm of permanent caval filtration. The decision whether the duration of protection is temporary or permanent should be made before insertion. The choice for transient caval filtration is based on the belief that the risk of complications from permanent caval filters is high, a concern that is based on observation and anecdotal experience. Considering that there are over 700 reports on the use of IVC filters during the past 35 years, it is disappointing that there is only one randomized trial evaluating efficacy of filters compared with anticoagulation in patients with established VTE[5-7] and one randomized comparative trial evaluating the outcomes of the Greenfield versus the TrapEase filters.[8]

Randomized trials

The PREPIC study[6,7] randomized 400 patients with proximal DVT who were at risk for PE to receive a vena caval filter or no filter in addition to routine anticoagulation. At day 12 and 12 months, patients in the filter group had lower rates of PE compared with the no filter group (1.1% vs. 4.8%), and after 2 years, symptomatic PE occurred in 3.4% of patients in the filter group versus 6.3% in the group without filters ($p = .16$). Recurrent DVT at 2 years, however, was greater in the filter group (20.8%) versus the group with no filter (11.6%; $p = .02$). The two groups demonstrated no difference in mortality or major bleeding.

At 8 years, the cumulative rate of symptomatic PE was 6.2% in the group with filters and 15.2% in those without filters ($p = .008$).[7] However, DVT occurred in 35.7 and 27.5% in the filter and no filter groups, respectively ($p = .042$). Postthrombotic syndrome and mortality were no different between the two groups.

The PREPIC study demonstrates that in patients who are candidates for anticoagulation, there is no survival benefit to having an IVC filter versus being treated with anticoagulation alone. Although there is a reduction in PE when a filter is inserted, it comes at a cost of increased risk of venous thrombosis. The PREPIC study group used a variety of filters. The relative outcomes following placement of IVC filters may well depend upon the filter used, as there are marked differences in vena caval filter hemodynamics and performance depending upon filter type.[9]

Usoh et al.[8] randomized 156 patients to receive either the stainless steel Greenfield filter or the TrapEase filter. Accepted indications for filter insertion were present in the majority of patients. During a mean 12-month follow-up, symptomatic vena caval thrombosis occurred in 5 patients (7%) in the TrapEase group and none in the Greenfield group (p = .19). Paradoxically, the Greenfield filter group may have been at higher risk for caval thrombosis, for they had a significantly higher proportion of patients with malignancy.

The observations from this randomized trial are consistent with the reports received by the U.S. Food and Drug Administration (FDA) MAUDE database.[10] The MAUDE database is composed of reports received by the FDA from manufacturers of device-related complications. Of the 724 Greenfield filters reported, 1.8% were associated with PE or an occluded vena cava, resulting in a death rate of 0.96%. The average time from filter insertion to the event was 11.4 days. There were 186 reports of the TrapEase or OptEase filter, of which 71 (36.2%) resulted in PE or IVC occlusion. The complications resulted in a death rate of 5.1%, and the average time from insertion to the event was 23 days.

Hemodynamic performance

A number of studies have been performed to evaluate the hemodynamics of several configurations of IVC filters. It is known that factors associated with thrombogenesis include: (1) turbulence, (2) near-wall velocity, and (3) wall shear stress.

Couch et al.[11] evaluated the hemodynamic characteristics of the 12 F titanium Greenfield and the Vena Tech LGM filters using an *in vitro* noninvasive flow visualization technique. Axial velocity profiles and wall shear stress distributions were measured. The results obtained with the filter in place were compared analytically to the flow field in the absence of the filter to determine the relative extent of the flow disturbances. The investigators found a marked reduction in near-wall axial velocity and wall shear stress in the Vena Tech filter compared with the Greenfield filter. These differences appeared to be the result of the geometry and dimensions of the struts attaching the filter

to the vena cava wall. Both filters demonstrated laminar flow fields without evidence of turbulence. The authors concluded that the reduced near-wall velocities and reduced wall shear stress in the Vena Tech LGM filter might increase the potential for thrombogenesis, and therefore caval occlusion, compared with the alternatively designed Greenfield filter.

Harlal et al.,[9] from the same laboratory, compared three IVC filters. The filters represented major design differences, which included (1) the inverted umbrella configuration (Mobin-Uddin filter [no longer available]), (2) the cone configuration (Greenfield filter), and (3) the combination of inverted umbrella and cone configurations (TrapEase/OptEase filters). The objective of this study was to identify the hemodynamics associated with each of these filters when no thrombus was present and when thrombus was trapped by the filter. The question was whether differences in hemodynamics could account for differences in filter performance, as observed from published clinical data.

The authors found that for both the open and partially occluded Mobin-Uddin and TrapEase filters, regions of flow stagnation or recirculation and turbulence developed downstream from the filter. The Greenfield filter did not produce any prothrombotic flow pattern for either the open or partially occluded filter. These performance results appear to correlate with published clinical studies indicating the increased thrombogenicity of the Mobin-Uddin and TrapEase filters compared with the Greenfield filter.

Decision matrix

The optimal therapy for VTE is pharmacologic and preventive.[1] There is no unique indication for the use of a nonpermanent filter, nor are there any evidence-based recommendations to support optional filters. Within the existing indications for filters, however, patients may have a limited period of risk for PE or a limited period of contraindication to anticoagulation.

Patients who have vena caval filters should be managed according to their venous thromboembolic status and their underlying condition. In other words, the presence of a filter does not mean the patient is "treated" for a PE or DVT. In the absence of a contraindication to anticoagulation, patients should be managed with appropriate anticoagulation. Currently, there is no absolute indication for filter retrieval, unless the filter itself is a source of major morbidity. Filter retrieval should occur only when the risk of PE is eliminated or minimal. The five fundamental considerations for use of an optional vena caval filter are (1) indication for placement, (2) management of the patient with the filter, (3) conditions for removal, (4) patient evaluation before removal, and (5) patient management after removal.

Indication for placement

If an indication for a permanent filter exists, a permanent filter should be inserted. A nonpermanent filter can be considered if the patient has a short, transient risk of PE, the patient does not have a venous thromboembolic complication and therefore the filter is truly prophylactic, or if the patient's duration of anticoagulation needs to be extended because of the filter. A suggested decision matrix regarding IVC filters is presented in Figure 9.1.

Management of the patient with a filter

All patients with an IVC filter should have optimal treatment for their underlying venous thromboembolic condition. Assuming the IVC filter was

placed because of a contraindication to anticoagulation, whenever the contraindication ends, anticoagulation should be initiated. If the patient is at high risk but VTE does not exist, the patient should receive optimal prophylaxis as soon as possible.

Hajduk et al.[12] performed a prospective observational cohort study of patients with vena caval filters who were subsequently anticoagulated after their contraindication to anticoagulation ended. In this cohort of 121 patients, symptomatic DVT subsequently developed in 24 patients (20%) and symptomatic PE in 6 patients (5%). What was unique about this study was the careful clinical surveillance and ongoing examinations of these patients. These patients underwent routine follow-up ultrasound examinations of their lower extremities and their inferior vena cavas. If nonocclusive thrombus was identified, in the filter or the leg, the patient's anticoagulation was increased; therefore, they underwent graded degrees of anticoagulation depending upon ultrasound findings. Only two episodes of occluded vena cavas were identified.

This approach is unique and may serve as a good comparison standard for future clinical trials, as well as an optimal method of management of patients with IVC filters.

Conditions for removal

Optional IVC filters can be considered for retrieval when the indication for the filter is no longer present and the patient is no longer at risk

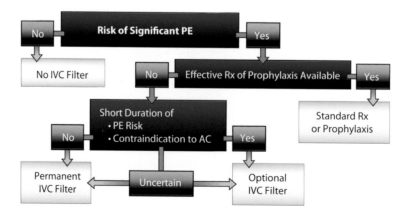

Figure 9.1 Decision matrix for the use of IVC filters.

for PE. Additionally, the patient should have a reasonable life expectancy and the return to a high risk for PE is unlikely. Patients should not have an underlying venous thromboembolic condition, or if they do, there should be no evidence of failure or complications of primary therapy. Furthermore, there should be no interval development of a venous thromboembolic complication since filter insertion.

Patient evaluation before removal

The goal of the patient evaluation before retrieval is to ensure that the risk of PE is low and that removal of the filter is safe. An algorithm for patient evaluation before retrieval is presented in Figure 9.2. Patients should routinely have a preintervention assessment for VTE risk and to determine whether interval DVT or PE has occurred. Their requirements for anticoagulation should be assessed, and if indicated, treatment should be ongoing and stable without duplex evidence of new thrombus formation. If anticoagulation is not required, the result of a venous duplex evaluation should be negative and imaging of the filter should not reveal unexpected findings.

Patient management after filter removal

Patients should be managed according to their underlying venous thromboembolic status and their underlying condition. Patients with VTE should receive anticoagulation according to established guidelines for therapy. A patient without venous thromboembolic complications should continue appropriate prophylaxis according to his or her underlying condition.

Summary

Unfortunately, reliable literature on IVC filters is sparse. In a recent basic data review on IVC filters,[13] 20 of 31 papers (65%) reporting an experience with retrievable IVC filters failed to report complications. Of 3052 retrievable filters reported, the average follow-up was 5.3 months and only 32% were retrieved. Therefore, until properly designed prospective studies are performed, treatment decisions are being based on opinion rather than data.

As mentioned previously, the hemodynamic performance of IVC filters varies with the

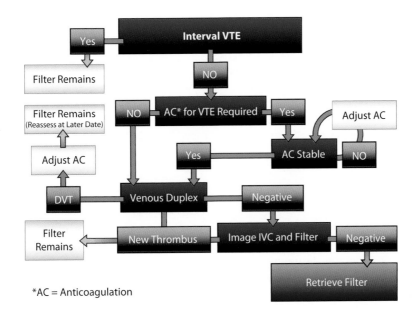

Figure 9.2 Decision matrix for removal of IVC filters.

filter configuration, impacting long-term outcome. There has been rapid acceptance of optional (retrievable) filters for use in trauma patients. Karmy-Jones et al.[14] reviewed practice patterns and outcomes of retrievable IVC filters in a large multicenter trauma study. Of 446 patients receiving IVC filters, 76% were placed for prophylactic indications. Only 22% of the filters were retrieved, and failed attempts at retrieval ranged from 10% to 27%, depending on filter type. Forty-six percent of the OptEase filter had significant thrombus versus 6% of the Günther-Tulip and 4% of the Bard-Recovery filter. Eleven percent of the OptEase filters resulted in caval occlusion compared with 1% and 0% of the Bard-Recovery and Günther-Tulip filters, respectively. Since the average follow-up in this series was 5.7 months, annualized parameters of thrombosis and caval occlusion would be more than double the reported outcomes.

These outcomes should be put into perspective of the long-term follow-up of trauma patients with permanent prophylactic IVC filters of the cone configuration. Phelan et al.[15] reported 188 patients receiving prophylactic vena caval filters. Fifty-two patients were followed for a mean of 8.8 years. There was no filter migration and no caval thrombosis; 1.5% had strut fracture, and 2% of the patients suffered a PE during follow-up. These data raise the question of whether there is any benefit of a contemporary retrievable filter compared to the permanent Greenfield filter.

It appears that the best patient outcomes will be delivered by physicians interested in the management of the problem of VTE, understanding that there may be transient risks to anticoagulation, that mechanical measures of prophylaxis may be used in patients with a transient risk of bleeding, and that filter design plays a crucial role in both short- and long-term complications.

REFERENCES

1. Kearon C, Kahn SR, Agnelli G, et al. Antithrombotic therapy for venous thromboembolic disease: ACCP evidence-based clinical practice guidelines (8th ed). *Chest* 2008; 133:454S–545S.

2. Passman MA. Vena caval interruption. In Cronenwett JL, Johnston W (eds.), *Rutherford's vascular surgery*. Philadelphia: Elsevier, 2010: 831–844.

3. Stein PD, Kayali F, Olson RE. Twenty-one-year trends in the use of inferior vena cava filters. *Arch Intern Med* 2004; 164:1541–1545.

4. Krishnamurthy VN, Greenfield LJ, Proctor MC, Rectenwald JE. Indications, techniques, and results of inferior vena cava filters. In Gloviczki P (ed.), *Handbook of venous disorders; guidelines of the American Venous Forum* (3rd ed.). London: Hodder, 2009: 299–313.

5. Girard P, Stern JB, Parent F. Medical literature and vena cava filters: so far so weak. *Chest* 2002; 122:963–967.

6. Decousus H, Leizorovicz A, Parent F, et al. A clinical trial of vena caval filters in the prevention of pulmonary embolism in patients with proximal deep-vein thrombosis. Prevention du Risque d'Embolie Pulmonaire par Interruption Cave Study Group. *N Engl J Med* 1998; 338:409–415.

7. Decousus H. Eight-year follow-up of a randomized trial investigating vena caval filters in the prevention of PE in patients presenting a proximal DVT: the PREPIC trial (abstract). *J Thromb Haemost* 2003; Suppl 11:OC440.

8. Usoh F, Hingorani A, Ascher E, et al. Prospective randomized study comparing the clinical outcomes between inferior vena cava Greenfield and TrapEase filters. *J Vasc Surg* 2010; 52:394–399.

9. Harlal A, Ojha M, Johnston KW. Vena cava filter performance based on hemodynamics and reported thrombosis and pulmonary embolism patterns. *J Vasc Interv Radiol* 2007; 18:103–115.

10. U.S. Department of Health and Human Services, Food and Drug Administration, Center for Devices and Radiological Health. *Guidance for cardiovascular intravascular filter submissions (510(k))*. Rockville, MD: Office of Device Evaluation, 2006.

11. Couch GG, Johnston KW, Ojha M. An *in vitro* comparison of the hemodynamics of two

inferior vena cava filters. *J Vasc Surg* 2000; 31:539–549.

12. Hajduk B, Tomkowski WZ, Malek G, Davidson BL. Vena cava filter occlusion and venous thromboembolism risk in persistently anti-coagulated patients: a prospective, observational cohort study. *Chest* 2010; 137:877–882.

13. Aziz F, Comerota AJ. Inferior vena cava filters. *Ann Vasc Surg* 2010; 24:966–979.

14. Karmy-Jones R, Jurkovich GJ, Velmahos GC, et al. Practice patterns and outcomes of retrievable vena cava filters in trauma patients: an AAST multicenter study. *J Trauma* 2007; 62:17–24.

15. Phelan HA, Gonzalez RP, Scott WC, et al. Long-term follow-up of trauma patients with permanent prophylactic vena cava filters. *J Trauma* 2009; 67:485–489.

10

Heparin-induced thrombocytopenia

Overview

Heparin-induced thrombocytopenia (HIT) is an immune-mediated coagulopathy caused by heparin-dependent antibodies resulting from heparin binding with platelet factor 4.[1] Early in the course of the recognition of HIT, vascular surgeons coined this disorder the "white clot syndrome," since the platelet fibrin thrombus causing the initial occlusion appeared white when removed from thrombosed arteries (Figures 10.1 and 10.2). HIT refers to the antibody-mediated coagulopathy most often associated with a significant drop in platelet clot. This is to be distinguished from the non-immune heparin-associated thrombocytopenia (HAT), which is observed to occur during heparin use that is not associated with antibody formation.[2] Despite the drop in platelet count, which can be severe, HIT is a thrombotic disorder, the complications of which are the result of thrombosis rather than bleeding. Studies have shown that 50% or more of patients with HIT will develop thrombosis if not properly treated.[1] The factors contributing to the prothrombotic state of HIT are listed in Box 10.1.

The frequency at which HIT occurs depends on several factors: the type of heparin, the type of patient, and duration of treatment. Bovine unfractionated heparin (UFH) has been associated with the greatest risk of HIT, followed by porcine UFH, followed by porcine low-molecular-weight heparin (LMWH). Fondaparinux generally is not associated with HIT, and only one case has been reported to date.[3] Some patients have higher risks than others. Surgical patients are generally at greater risk than are medical patients, who are at greater risk

than obstetrical patients. Of the surgical patients, orthopedic patients and patients undergoing coronary artery bypass are at greatest risk.

The longer the duration of administration, the more likely HIT is to occur, and hence the necessity of monitoring platelet counts. Prior exposure to heparin may predispose the patient to a rapid fall in platelet count upon reexposure because of existing antibodies. This is the typical presentation of patients who develop HIT when administered heparin intraoperatively, as these patients have had exposure to UFH in the recent past and have high titers of heparin antibodies.

An unusual form of HIT can begin several days after heparin has been discontinued. This is known as delayed-onset HIT.[4] This occurs as a result of high-titer HIT antibodies, which are capable of activating platelets in the absence of heparin.[5]

Clinical presentation

HIT can develop in patients receiving low doses of heparin subcutaneously or by continuous infusion. There is no specific dose relationship, and HIT has been observed in patients receiving only heparin flushes or who have heparin-coated indwelling catheters.

In general, patients develop HIT after receiving UFH for a period of 5 to 10 days or more. As mentioned previously, a rapid drop in platelet count can occur in patients with recent exposure who have established antibodies.[6–8]

HIT is a dangerous prothrombotic state that can cause life- or limb-threatening thromboses.

BOX 10.1 FACTORS CONTRIBUTING TO THE PROTHROMBOTIC STATE OF HIT

1. Platelet activation
2. Monocyte activation
3. Endothelial dysfunction
4. Increased tissue factor
5. Platelet and leukocyte binding to endothelium
6. Platelet-derived microparticles
7. PF4 neutralization of heparin
8. Increased thrombin generation

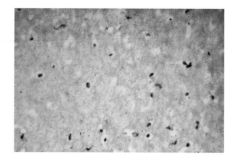

Figure 10.2 Hematoxylin–eosin (H&E) stain of "white clot" showing only fibrin and platelets.

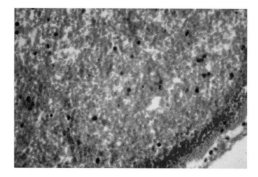

Figure 10.3 H&E stain of normal thrombus showing predominance of red blood cells.

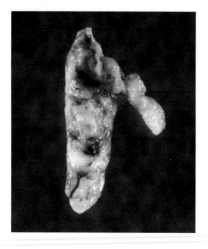

Figure 10.1 "White clot" removed from an acutely thrombosed femoral bifurcation in a patient developing HIT after receiving heparin infusion following a contralateral femoropopliteal bypass. Note the cast of the femoral bifurcation, which outlines the distal common femoral and proximal superficial femoral arteries and origin of the profunda femoris artery. The patient developed profound limb ischemia at the time of arterial occlusion.

Early observational and natural history studies have documented that up to 50% of patients develop thrombosis in the absence of adequate treatment.[9,10] Venous thromboembolic complications are the most common with HIT. However, arterial thrombotic events are frequently observed in patients who have been treated for atherosclerotic complications of their arterial disease (Figures 10.1–10.3). Acute arterial thrombotic complications often present as acute ischemia in all vascular beds, coronary, cerebrovascular, and peripheral.

Heparin-induced skin necrosis can occur and is observed when heparin is injected subcutaneously in patients with established antibodies.

Diagnosis

Diagnosis of HIT is based on both clinical criteria, which are the development of thrombocytopenia or thrombotic events while patients are receiving heparin, and laboratory data (platelet count and HIT antibodies).

It has been observed that the severity of the induced thrombocytopenia is a good predictor of additional thromboses and amputation.[11] Platelet counts should be monitored in all patients on heparin and should be performed every other day in patients considered at high risk and every 2 to 3 days in patients considered intermediate risk, beginning on day 4 and extending to at least day 14.[12] HIT should be suspected if the platelet count drops to <150,000 or there is a ≥50% drop occurring during heparin administration.

Unexplained thrombosis that occurs during or after a recent heparin administration, even in the absence of thrombocytopenia, should raise the suspicion of a heparin-induced prothrombotic state, as the absence of a low platelet count does not exclude HIT.

The two major categories of assays are platelet activation tests (i.e., serotonin release assay) and antigen assays (i.e., enzyme-linked immunosorbent assay [ELISA]).

The serotonin release assay that detects HIT antibody-induced platelet activation is considered the most reliable laboratory test. Plasma or serum of the patient suspected of HIT is obtained and mixed with washed donor platelets, which are loaded with 14C-serotonin in the presence of low doses and high doses of heparin. Anti-PF4 (platelet factor 4) antibodies cause platelet activation, resulting in high 14C-serotonin levels, which are released from the platelet granules as a result of low-dose heparin exposure. This reaction does not occur in the presence of high concentrations of heparin due to supersaturation of the antibodies. A positive result is diagnostic of HIT.

The ELISA antigen assays are generally performed with commercial kits. These assays are highly sensitive and have a high negative predictive value; however, many tests can be false-positive. In difficult clinical situations, if the ELISA antigen assay and the serotonin release assay are positive, the diagnosis of HIT is essentially confirmed. Likewise, if both tests are negative, HIT is excluded. If these tests disagree, the serotonin release assay is considered the more reliable laboratory test supporting or excluding the diagnosis of HIT.

Management

When HIT is suspected, all forms of heparin should be discontinued. Even heparin flushes, heparin-coated catheters, and heparin-bonded grafts should be avoided. Table 10.1 lists key American College of Chest Physicians (ACCP) guidelines for HIT.

Because of the high risk of thrombosis developing in nontreated patients, the diagnosis of HIT mandates therapy.[12] As mentioned before, HIT

Table 10.1 Key ACCP recommendations for HIT

Recommendation	Grade
In all patients with suspected HIT, heparin compounds should be discontinued and diagnostic testing instituted.	1B
For patients with suspected HIT, treatment with a nonheparin anticoagulant such as argatroban, lepirudin, bivalirudin, danaparoid, or fondaparinux should be instituted.	1B
VKAs should be avoided until the platelet count returns to near normal.	1B
For patients receiving a VKA at the time of the diagnosis of HIT, vitamin K should be given to reverse the anticoagulant effect.	1C
For patients with strongly suspected or confirmed HIT, routine ultrasonography of the lower-extremity veins should be performed.	1C
Prophylactic platelet transfusions should be avoided.	1C
Patients receiving heparin should have platelet count monitoring.	1C
In patients who have received heparin within the past 3 months and who are about to begin heparin therapy, a baseline platelet count should be obtained, followed by a repeat platelet count 24 hours after heparin is restarted.	1C
In patients receiving heparin whose platelet count drops to 50% of baseline platelet count or less than 150,000, HIT should be suspected.	2C

Source: Warkentin TE, et al., *Chest* 2008; 133:340S–380S.

Note: ACCP, American College of Chest Physicians; HIT, heparin-induced thrombocytopenia; VKA, vitamin K antagonist.

is a strongly prothrombotic state associated with thrombin generation. As such, direct thrombin inhibitors have been useful in the management of patients with HIT. The reader is referred to Chapter 5 for additional details, although the basic summary of treatment will follow.

Lepirudin

Lepirudin is a recombinant hirudin that irreversibly binds directly to thrombin. Its intravenous half-life is 60 to 80 minutes and should be avoided in patients with compromised renal function. Lepirudin is monitored by the activated partial thromboplastin time (aPTT) after being infused at a dose of 0.05 to 0.10 mg/kg/hr, with a target aPTT of 2× control. Patients presenting with an acute thrombotic complication should receive a bolus dose of 0.2 to 0.4 mg/kg.

Bivalirudin

Bivalirudin is a variant of hirudin, as it contains two short synthetic hirudin peptide fragments having a half-life of 25 minutes. Bivalirudin is administered intravenously at a dose of 0.15 mg/kg/hr to a target aPTT of 1.5 to 2.5× baseline.

Argatroban

Argatroban is a synthetic direct thrombin inhibitor metabolized by the liver with a half-life of 45 minutes. Argatroban is administered intravenously with an initial infusion rate of 2 mcg/kg/min, which is reduced as the aPTT is monitored. The dose is generally adjusted to maintain the aPTT to 1.5 to 3.0× control.

Danaparoid

While danaparoid is not available in the United States, it is often the first-line therapy for HIT in Europe, Australia, and New Zealand. Danaparoid is infused intravenously at a bolus of 2250 units followed by 400 U/hr for 4 hours, 300 U/hr for 4 hours, and then 200 U/hr for 5 days or longer.

Fondaparinux

Although fondaparinux is not approved for management of patients with HIT, it has been used in this clinical situation. Its excellent bioavailability and half-life of 17 to 20 hours allow once-per-day subcutaneous dosing. Fondaparinux is used therapeutically at a dose of 7.5 mg daily for patients weighing 50 to 100 kg. The dose is decreased to 5 mg daily for patients weighing less than 50 kg and increased to 10 mg daily for those weighing more than 100 kg.

Other management

Since HIT is a strong prothrombotic state and since warfarin also produces a prothrombotic state early in the course of therapy, warfarin is contraindicated during the initial treatment of HIT. Patients treated early in the course of HIT with VKAs face a risk of the serious complication of warfarin-induced skin necrosis (Figure 10.4). If long-term anticoagulation for the patient's underlying thrombotic disorder is indicated and warfarin is to be used, its initiation should be delayed until the platelet count has returned to near-normal levels. At this point, VKAs can be started at low doses and gradually increased. If warfarin was already initiated prior to the diagnosis of HIT, physicians should consider neutralizing its effect with vitamin K.

The duration of treatment with the direct thrombin inhibitors should be continued at least until the platelet count returns to normal. At that point the decision is made whether ongoing anticoagulation is appropriate, depending upon the patient's initial and persistent indication for anticoagulation.

Platelet transfusions should be avoided in patients with HIT, despite low platelet counts, since circulating antibodies in the plasma bind to the transfused platelets and additional platelet activation and aggregation occur.

Patients being evaluated for the implantation of a heparin-bonded prosthetic should undergo preoperative testing for heparin platelet factor 4 (PF4) antibodies to reduce the risk of HIT postimplantation. HIT has been reported after implantation of a heparin-bonded polytetrafluoroethylene (PTFE) lower-extremity bypass,[13] and the plan for management of patients being considered for heparin-bonded implants is reviewed in Figure 10.5.

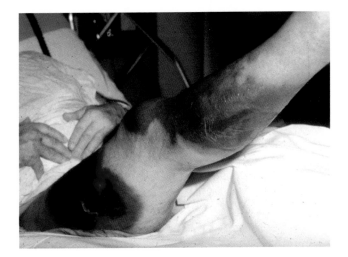

Figure 10.4 Vitamin K-induced skin necrosis in the lower limb of a patient started on warfarin early after the diagnosis of HIT.

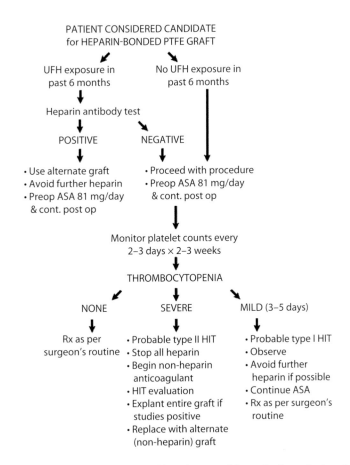

Figure 10.5 Suggested protocol for patients considered as candidates for heparin-bonded prosthesis.

REFERENCES

1. Warkentin TE. Heparin-induced thrombocytopenia: pathogenesis and management. *Br J Haematol* 2003; 121:535–555.
2. Chong BH. Heparin-induced thrombocytopenia. *J Thromb Haemost* 2003; 1:1471–1478.
3. Warkentin TE. Heparin-induced thrombocytopenia associated with fondaparinux. *N Engl J Med* 2007; 356:2653–2654.
4. Rice L, Attisha WK, Drexler A, Francis JL. Delayed-onset heparin-induced thrombocytopenia. *Ann Intern Med* 2002; 136:210–215.
5. Warkentin TE, Kelton JG. Delayed-onset heparin-induced thrombocytopenia and thrombosis. *Ann Intern Med* 2001; 135: 502–506.
6. Warkentin TE, Kelton JG. Temporal aspects of heparin-induced thrombocytopenia. *N Engl J Med* 2001; 344:1286–1292.
7. Chong BH, Fawaz I, Chesterman CN, Berndt MC. Heparin-induced thrombocytopenia: mechanism of interaction of the heparin-dependent antibody with platelets. *Br J Haematol* 1989; 73:235–240.
8. Chong BH, Grace CS, Rozenberg MC. Heparin-induced thrombocytopenia: effect of heparin platelet antibody on platelets. *Br J Haematol* 1981; 49:531–540.
9. Warkentin TE, Kelton JG. A 14-year study of heparin-induced thrombocytopenia. *Am J Med* 1996; 101:502–507.
10. Hirsh J, Heddle N, Kelton JG. Treatment of heparin-induced thrombocytopenia: a critical review. *Arch Intern Med* 2004; 164: 361–369.
11. Kelton JG, Hursting MJ, Heddle N, Lewis BE. Predictors of clinical outcome in patients with heparin-induced thrombocytopenia treated with direct thrombin inhibition. *Blood Coagul Fibrinolysis* 2008; 19:471–475.
12. Warkentin TE, Greinacher A, Koster A, Lincoff AM. Treatment and prevention of heparin-induced thrombocytopenia: American College of Chest Physicians Evidence-Based Clinical Practice Guidelines (8th edition). *Chest* 2008; 133:340S–380S.
13. Thakur S, Pigott JP, Comerota AJ. Heparin-induced thrombocytopenia after implantation of a heparin-bonded polytetrafluoroethylene lower extremity bypass graft: a case report and plan for management. *J Vasc Surg* 2009; 49:1037–1040.

Common femoral endovenectomy and endoluminal recanalization for chronic postthrombotic iliofemoral venous obstruction

Overview

Natural history studies of anticoagulation for iliofemoral deep venous thrombosis (DVT) treated with anticoagulation alone have shown that, at 5 years, over 90% of patients have venous insufficiency, 15% have experienced venous ulceration, and up to 50% have compromised ambulation as a result of the discomfort of ambulatory venous hypertension.[1,2] Patients with chronic postthrombotic iliofemoral venous obstruction have a significantly reduced quality of life, which could have been avoided if their acute DVT had been treated with a strategy of thrombus removal.[3] A prospective observational study has shown that iliofemoral DVT patients have the most severe postthrombotic morbidity.[4] Unfortunately, most patients are treated with anticoagulation alone rather than a strategy of thrombus removal, as many physicians fail to appreciate the connection between iliofemoral venous obstruction and the subsequent severity of postthrombotic morbidity.

The pathophysiology of postthrombotic venous insufficiency is ambulatory venous hypertension, which is defined as elevated venous pressures during exercise[5,6] and is particularly severe when valvular incompetence and venous obstruction coexist. While valvular function can be quantified

through ultrasonography, residual venous obstruction frequently goes undetected, as it adversely affects venous hemodynamics but is difficult to image and impossible to quantify. Unfortunately, lower-extremity venous outflow studies, which are the basis to noninvasively detect venous outflow obstruction, are notoriously inadequate in identifying iliac venous obstruction or occlusion. This inability to noninvasively quantitate venous obstruction has led to a widespread underappreciation of its contribution to postthrombotic morbidity. Labropoulos et al.[7] measured venous pressure gradients across the spectrum of patients with postthrombotic venous disease and normal controls and found that chronic iliofemoral venous occlusion was associated with the highest resting and exercise venous pressure gradients.

Patients with postthrombotic obstruction isolated to the iliac veins often can be successfully treated with angioplasty and stenting alone,[8,9] but if the chronic occlusive disease includes the common femoral vein (CFV), treatment is more challenging. Following percutaneous intervention, relative obstruction of the CFV can persist, leading to incomplete drainage of the femoral and profunda femoris venous systems, thereby mitigating the benefit of iliac vein recanalization. Although stenting across the inguinal ligament can be performed, the risk of stent occlusion is increased in postthrombotic patients.[8] Moreover, personal observations have demonstrated that when a CFV stent compromises drainage from the profunda femoris vein, the patient's clinical status can worsen. Based upon these observations, it seems appropriate to surgically eliminate the CFV obstruction and endoluminally recanalize the obstructed iliocaval segments.

The procedure described in this chapter is indicated for patients with chronic postthrombotic iliofemoral venous obstruction causing severe postthrombotic syndrome and in whom the CFV is badly diseased. The goal of the procedure is to provide unobstructed venous drainage from the profunda femoris vein to the vena cava. As many of these patients have severe residual postthrombotic obstruction or occlusion of the femoral vein, the profunda femoris represents the major venous drainage from the infrainguinal venous system. To date, we have treated 16 patients with severe postthrombotic iliofemoral/vena caval venous obstruction presenting with clinical class C3–C6 of the clinical, etiologic, anatomic, pathophysiologic (CEAP) classification. The duration of their obstruction ranged from 7 months to 20 years (mean 6.8 years).

Operative procedure

Preoperative evaluation includes a complete noninvasive evaluation, which includes a venous duplex (Figure 11.1), venous physiologic studies bilaterally, and a complete phlebography of the target leg, including the inferior vena cava, to document the extent of the patient's venous obstruction (Figure 11.2).[10] A guidewire is maneuvered through the obstructed venous segments during the preoperative venogram to ensure that passage through the occluded venous segments can be achieved and recanalization can be accomplished in the operating room. Two to three days prior to the operative procedure, patients are started on combined platelet inhibition with aspirin (81 mg/day) and clopidogrel (75 mg/day). Chlorhexidine showers twice daily are implemented and vitamin K antagonists (VKAs) discontinued.

The CFV, distal external iliac vein, cephalad portion of the femoral vein, and profunda femoris vein are exposed through a standard longitudinal inguinal incision (Figure 11.3). Control of all branches, especially posterior CFV branches, is obtained. Small tributaries are ligated or controlled with surgical clips. Patients are fully anticoagulated with 100 IU/kg of unfractionated heparin (UFH). A longitudinal venotomy is then performed that often incorporates the proximal femoral vein to the distal external iliac vein (Figures 11.4a, b). Dense fibrinous tissue and web-like synechiae are removed with sharp and blunt dissection extended into the distal external iliac vein (Figure 11.5a). Careful attention is given to the orifice of the profunda femoris vein(s) (Figure 11.5b). In most patients, sharp excision is required, usually with small angled scissors, as the fibrous evolution of thrombus forms dense adherence to the vein wall. One can generally get an impression as to the proper plane, although the endovenectomy is unlike an arterial endarterectomy, where the atherosclerotic plaque cleanly peels away from the vessel wall, leaving a smooth arterial wall. Patch closure of the venotomy is performed using bovine pericardium (Figure 11.6) or saphenous vein, leaving the caudal centimeter open to introduce a 10 Fr sheath (Figure 11.7a) through which the endoluminal recanalization of the iliac venous segment is performed.

A separate stab incision is made below the inguinal wound through which the sheath is passed, traversing the subcutaneous tissue, and enters the CFV without angulation (Figure 11.7b). A vascular tourniquet placed around the distal CFV

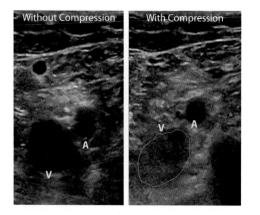

Figure 11.1 Preoperative venous duplex (left) shows noncompressed common femoral vein (V) and artery (A); right frame illustrates that the common femoral vein is noncompressible due to extensive intraluminal fibrosis.

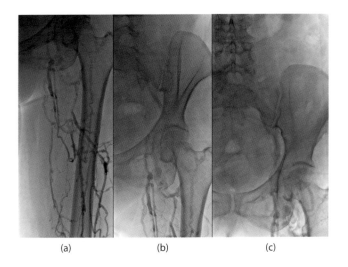

(a)   (b)   (c)

Figure 11.2 (a–c) Preoperative venogram demonstrates extensive venous obstruction from the mid-thigh to the vena cava in a patient incapacitated following iliofemoral and femoropopliteal DVT 7 months earlier. The patient was hospitalized and treated for recurrent acute iliofemoral DVT 2 months earlier. (From Vogel D, et al., *J Vasc Surg* 2012; 55(1):129–135. Reprinted with permission from Elsevier.)

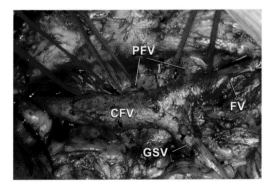

Figure 11.3 Operative exposure of the common femoral vein (CFV), femoral vein (FV), saphenofemoral junction (SFJ), and origins of the profunda femoris veins (PFVs). Smaller tributaries are ligated or controlled with vessel loops. Dissection is extended cephalad to under the inguinal ligament exposing the distal external iliac vein (EIV). (From Vogel D, et al., *J Vasc Surg* 2012; 55(1):129–135. Reprinted with permission from Elsevier.)

secures the sheath. All clamps are left in place to limit the amount of stagnant blood in contact with the thrombogenic vein wall and sheath. After the guidewire is passed into the patent inferior vena cava (IVC), the iliac venous system and, if necessary, vena cava are sequentially recanalized with balloon dilation and subsequent stenting (Figure 11.8). In

general, Wallstents are preferred because of their high radial strength (resistance to compression), with 14 to 18 mm stents used for the common iliac veins and 12 to 14 mm for the external iliac veins. Stents are extended partially into the IVC, only to fully treat the common iliac lesion. Stents may be brought below the inguinal ligament into the endo-venectomized CFV. We always terminate the stent above the saphenofemoral junction to ensure that there is no compromise of drainage from the profunda femoris vein. External iliac stents are placed initially, followed by stenting of the common iliac vein. If IVC stents are required, they will be placed first. Stents are postdilated to their target diameter. We have found intravascular ultrasound (IVUS) valuable in assessing the limits of the procedure and final result, and IVUS is now used routinely.

Following recanalization and venographic confirmation of unobstructed venous drainage from the CFV to the IVC, the sheath is removed and closure of the patch venoplasty is completed (Figure 11.9). A 7F silastic closed suction drain is brought through the stab wound used for the sheath and maintained on suction postoperatively until drainage volume is less than 20 cc/12 hr. The incision is closed with several layers of running absorbable suture, obliterating dead space and ensuring lymphostatic and hemostatic closure of the subcutaneous tissue.

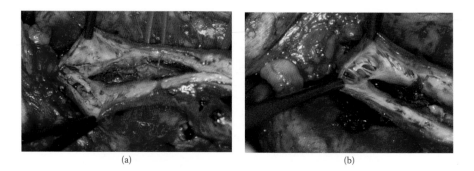

(a) (b)

Figure 11.4 (a) A longitudinal venotomy often incorporates the distal external iliac vein to the proximal femoral vein. Fibrotic transformation of occlusive thrombus is observed adherent to the vein wall with a remaining core of 2-month-old thrombus. This patient had her initial iliofemoral DVT 7 months earlier and experienced recurrent acute DVT 2.5 months prior to the operation. (b) Distal external iliac vein with characteristic fibrous webs and synechiae. (From Vogel D, et al., *J Vasc Surg* 2012; 55(1):129–135. Reprinted with permission from Elsevier.)

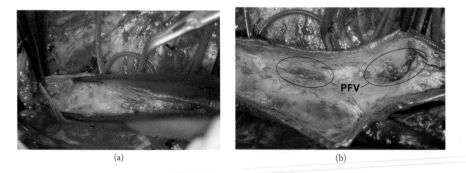

(a) (b)

Figure 11.5 (a) Post endovenectomy, the distal external iliac and the common femoral vein are cleared of obstruction, (b) with the dissection extending into the orifice(s) of the profunda venous system. (From Vogel D, et al., *J Vasc Surg* 2012; 55(1):129–135. Reprinted with permission from Elsevier.)

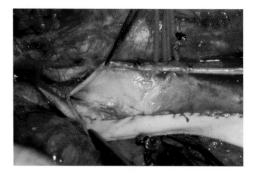

Figure 11.6 Patch closure of the common femoral vein following endovenectomy. Patch is bovine pericardium.

Heparin is not reversed with protamine. In some patients, a silastic intravenous catheter was placed in a dorsal foot vein to infuse postoperative heparin; the intent was to achieve high concentrations of heparin in the treated veins while reducing the need for high systemic doses of anticoagulation. The remainder received standard intravenous therapeutic UFH infusion. The CFV is examined with a continuous-wave Doppler after clamps are removed. If robust venous velocity signals are not present, a small arteriovenous fistula (AVF) is constructed (Figure 11.10). At the present time, I believe it is prudent to construct a small distal AVF in all patients.

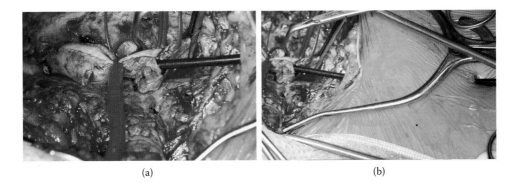

(a)   (b)

Figure 11.7 (a) Caudal end of patch closure is left open to advance a 10F sheath secured by a vascular tourniquet, which was (b) brought into the wound through a separate stab incision in the thigh.

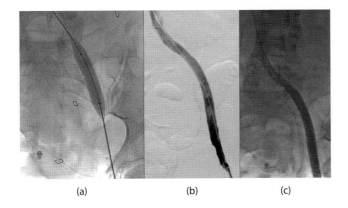

(a)   (b)   (c)

Figure 11.8 (a) Following guidewire passage into the patent IVC, a balloon catheter is passed and preliminary balloon dilation is performed. (b) Stenting of the occluded external iliac and common iliac veins is completed, and (c) an intraoperative completion phlebogram is performed to document unobstructed venous flow into the IVC.

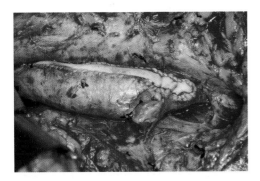

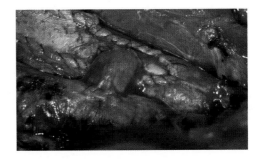

Figure 11.9 Following removal of the sheath, closure of the patch venoplasty is completed. The proximal femoral and saphenous veins were resected. Picture shows CFV patch extending onto the PFV.

Figure 11.10 A small arteriovenous fistula is constructed from the superficial femoral artery (SFA) to the distal common femoral vein patch using a saphenous interposition graft.

Patients are anticoagulated postoperatively with unfractionated heparin converted to warfarin. Since most patients have had recurrent DVT, indefinite anticoagulation is planned. Clopidogrel is discontinued at 8 weeks postoperatively; however, aspirin is continued at 81 mg/day.

Operative complications

In our series to date, one operative mortality has occurred: a patient died 9 days after discharge from an acute myocardial infarction. Three patients developed wound hematomas requiring operative evacuation, and three developed early postoperative thrombosis. All recurrent thromboses were treated, and all patients were discharged with patent reconstructions. One patient who had a nonhealing venous ulcer developed a chronic wound infection and acute postoperative lymphedema.

Clinical outcomes

Preoperative and postoperative evaluations are performed using the Venous Clinical Severity Score (VCSS), the Villalta scale, the clinical classification of CEAP, and completion of the validated VEINES-QOL/Sym questionnaire.

The VCSS identifies 10 clinical characteristics of chronic venous disease that are graded from 0 to 3 (absent, mild, moderate, severe) with specific criteria to avoid overlap or arbitrary scoring.[11] The Villalta scale consists of six clinician-rated physical signs and five patient-rated venous symptoms, of which each are rated on a 4-point scale (0 = none, 1 = mild, 2 = moderate, 3 = severe). Points are summed to produce a total score (range 0–33). Subjects are classified as having postthrombotic syndrome (PTS) if the score is ≥5 or if a venous ulcer is present in a leg with previous DVT. The Villalta scale is a validated, reliable method of identifying patients with the postthrombotic syndrome.[12]

The CEAP clinical classification is based on a 7-point clinical assessment of venous disease.[13] The anatomical distribution of venous obstruction included the CFV and iliac venous segments in all patients. The VEINES-QOL/Sym questionnaire is a tool designed to assess quality of life (QOL) and symptoms of chronic venous insufficiency[14,15]

and is modeled after the SF-36. All patients are followed at 3, 6, and 12 months and every 6 months thereafter.

In our cohort of patients, all clinical outcome measurements improved following endovenectomy and iliac recanalization (mean follow-up 8.8 months). The mean preoperative VCSS of 17 dropped to 10 postoperatively ($p = .02$). Villalta scores improved from a mean of 14 preoperatively to 6 ($p = .002$). Overall QOL and symptoms improved as assessed by VEINES-QOL/Sym ($p = .01$ and .02, respectively). Preoperative CEAP scores in the study patients ranged from C4 (pigmentation changes, venous eczema, lipodermatosclerosis) to C5 (healed venous stasis ulceration) and C6 (active venous stasis ulceration). Three patients with preoperative ulcers had a CEAP classification change from 6 to 5 due to their ulcers healing postendovenectomy and iliocaval recanalization. The remaining patients who had preoperative CEAP scores of 4 or 5 demonstrated improvement in their symptoms.

Ultrasound evaluation at follow-up showed one segmental occlusion of the CFV; however, the patient was improved compared to preoperative status. The remaining patients continue to have patent veins.

Perspective

Common femoral endovenectomy with endoluminal iliac vein recanalization is a promising treatment to eliminate proximal venous obstruction and reduce incapacitating postthrombotic morbidity. Since the iliofemoral venous segment is the single venous outflow channel from the leg, it is understandable that obstruction of this segment causes incapacitating morbidity.

As observed in our patient cohort, this procedure has the potential of substantially improving patient function and quality of life. Although the technical details have been previously reported,[16] several key elements are worth emphasizing. Complete control of all branches of the CFV is mandatory, as endovenectomy must be performed in a completely dry field. Ensuring unobstructed venous drainage from the profunda femoris vein into the patent vena cava is mandatory. Although IVUS was not used early in our experience, we have found it to be a valuable adjunct. We may have averted one of our early postoperative thromboses if IVUS had been used during the procedure. Therefore, its use is now routine.

The construction of an adjunctive AVF was not performed in some cases because of the robust venous velocity signals obtained when the procedure was completed. However, aggressive anticoagulation with combined platelet inhibition led to a return to the operating room for evacuation of wound hematomas in three patients, which might have been avoided if AVFs had been constructed and less intense anticoagulation used.

Endovenectomy (or endophlebectomy) has been an infrequently reported procedure for venous obstruction. Early reports of removing obstruction from the superior vena cava[17-19] were followed by the case report of Breslau and DeWeese,[20] who described successful treatment of an occluded saphenous vein functioning as a bypass graft. Gloviczki and Cho[21] suggested that CFV endovenectomy could be performed, and Puggioni et al.[22] reported that segmental endovenectomy could be performed as part of a venous reconstructive procedure. More recently, Garg et al.[23] described outcomes of 12 patients who underwent CFV endovenectomy, patch angioplasty, and stenting for chronic iliofemoral venous obstruction. They reported rather pessimistic results, which contrast with our observations thus far.

Iliac venous stenting has become the method of choice for correcting iliac venous obstruction.[24] Iliac stenting has for the most part been successful, with primary, assisted-primary, and secondary patency rates of 57%, 80%, and 86%, respectively, in postthrombotic patients, with low complication rates.[8] However, if the stent is extended below the inguinal ligament, there is at least a 3.8-fold risk of stent occlusion in postthrombotic limbs.[8,25] Despite the increased risk of occlusion, many postthrombotic patients require stenting into the CFV to adequately treat skip lesions and areas of residual stenosis that, if left untreated, might lead to recurrent thrombosis.[26,27] We believe that many of the failures in these patients are due to residual and underappreciated obstructive disease in the CFV.

As noted by Raju et al.,[26,27] postthrombotic limbs are at a higher risk of recurrent occlusion following iliac vein stenting (82% vs. 100% 5-year patency in nonthrombotic iliac vein lesions [NIVLs]).

Based upon personal experience, stenting into the distal CFV and potentially restricting drainage from the orifice of the profunda femoris vein in a postthrombotic CFV can lead to further compromise of venous outflow as a result of the stent compressing a fibrous flap across the profunda's orifice. When this occurs, there is notable progression of obstructive symptoms, with increasing edema, pain, and venous claudication.

Chronic central venous obstruction was the overriding pathology in our patients. Although all of our patients also had infrainguinal postthrombotic venous disease with damaged valves, their severe disability resulted from their iliofemoral/caval obstruction. Lugli and Maleti[28,29] reported constructing a neovalve in the femoral vein of patients with postthrombotic syndrome. The neovalve was constructed in patients without proximal obstruction, which is a different subset of patients than reported here. We did not perform any intervention below the common femoral vein, although ligation and resection of the femoral vein were performed when it was severely obstructed or occluded.

By performing a hybrid procedure of open endovenectomy and endoluminal iliac recanalization, several important anatomical derangements can be corrected. First, the profunda femoris orifices can be disobliterated, thus allowing maximal drainage from the thigh and lower leg. Second, the multiple recanalization channels of outflow from dense fibrinous tissue with the synechiae in the CFV or CFV occlusions are cleared into the distal external iliac vein. Once completed, the iliac venous stenosis or occlusion can be stented into the endovenectomized portion of the external iliac vein or CFV, ensuring unobstructed flow to the inferior vena cava. This approach avoids skip lesions that might otherwise lead to reocclusion or continued functional compromise. While we attempted to keep stents above the inguinal ligament early in our experience, we now believe it is reasonable to extend the stents below the inguinal ligament into the endovenectomized CFV if necessary; however, we believe it is imperative to keep the distal end of the stent above the saphenofemoral junction to ensure preservation of profunda femoris venous drainage. In several patients with severe disease of the femoral vein, it was ligated and the cephalad femoral vein resected. Occluded and incompetent saphenous veins are also ligated, and that portion of vein exposed within the incision is resected.

This procedure has resulted in remarkable improvement in the clinical signs and symptoms of the postthrombotic syndrome in patients followed up to 36 months. No patients have clinically or physiologically deteriorated following their objective outcome assessment. Postoperative morbidity was acceptable, although with refinement of the technique as experience is gained, less operative morbidity should be expected. All patients returned to full daily activity, including employment for those not retired. All three patients with long-standing venous ulcers healed without need for further intervention.

Conclusion

Common femoral endovenectomy with iliocaval endoluminal recanalization is a safe and promising procedure for patients with chronic extensive postthrombotic iliofemoral/vena caval venous obstruction. It restores unobstructed venous drainage from the profunda femoris vein to the vena cava, resulting in improved quality of life and reduced postthrombotic morbidity.

REFERENCES

1. Akesson H, Brudin L, Dahlstrom JA, Eklof B, Ohlin P, Plate G. Venous function assessed during a 5 year period after acute ilio-femoral venous thrombosis treated with anticoagulation. *Eur J Vasc Surg* 1990; 4:43–48.

2. Delis KT, Bountouroglou D, Mansfield AO. Venous claudication in iliofemoral thrombosis: long-term effects on venous hemodynamics, clinical status, and quality of life. *Ann Surg* 2004; 239:118–126.

3. Comerota AJ, Throm RC, Mathias SD, Haughton S, Mewissen M. Catheter-directed thrombolysis for iliofemoral deep venous thrombosis improves health-related quality of life. *J Vasc Surg* 2000; 32:130–137.

4. Kahn SR, Shrier I, Julian JA, et al. Determinants and time course of the postthrombotic syndrome after acute deep venous thrombosis. *Ann Intern Med* 2008; 149:698–707.

5. Shull KC, Nicolaides AN, Fernandes e Fernandes J, et al. Significance of popliteal reflux in relation to ambulatory venous pressure and ulceration. *Arch Surg* 1979; 114:1304–1306.

6. Nicolaides AN, Schull K, Fernandes E. Ambulatory venous pressure: new information. In Nicolaides AN, Yao JS (eds.), *Investigation of vascular disorders*. New York: Churchill Livingstone, 1981: 488–494.

7. Labropoulos N, Volteas N, Leon M, et al. The role of venous outflow obstruction in patients with chronic venous dysfunction. *Arch Surg* 1997; 132:46–51.

8. Neglen P, Hollis KC, Olivier J, Raju S. Stenting of the venous outflow in chronic venous disease: long-term stent-related outcome, clinical, and hemodynamic result. *J Vasc Surg* 2007; 46:979–990.

9. Kolbel T, Lindh M, Akesson M, Wasselius J, Gottsater A, Ivancev K. Chronic iliac vein occlusion: midterm results of endovascular recanalization. *J Endovasc Ther* 2009; 16:483–491.

10. Vogel D, Comerota AJ, Al-Jabouri, M, Assi, ZI. Common femoral endovenectomy with iliocaval endoluminal recanalization improves symptoms and quality of life in patients with postthrombotic iliofemoral obstruction. *J Vasc Surg* 2012; 55(1): 129–135.

11. Rutherford RB, Padberg FT Jr., Comerota AJ, Kistner RL, Meissner MH, Moneta GL. Venous severity scoring: an adjunct to venous outcome assessment. *J Vasc Surg* 2000; 31:1307–1312.

12. Kahn SR. Measurement properties of the Villalta scale to define and classify the severity of the post-thrombotic syndrome. *J Thromb Haemost* 2009; 7:884–888.

13. Eklof B, Rutherford RB, Bergan JJ, et al. Revision of the CEAP classification for chronic venous disorders: consensus statement. *J Vasc Surg* 2004; 40:1248–1252.

14. Kahn SR, Lamping DL, Ducruet T, et al. VEINES-QOL/Sym questionnaire was a reliable and valid disease-specific quality of life measure for deep venous thrombosis. *J Clin Epidemiol* 2006; 59:1049–1056.

15. Lamping DL, Schroter S, Kurz X, Kahn SR, Abenhaim L. Evaluation of outcomes in chronic venous disorders of the leg:

development of a scientifically rigorous, patient-reported measure of symptoms and quality of life. *J Vasc Surg* 2003; 37:410–419.

16. Comerota AJ, Grewal NK, Thakur S, Assi Z. Endovenectomy of the common femoral vein and intraoperative iliac vein recanalization for chronic iliofemoral venous occlusion. *J Vasc Surg* 2010; 52:243–247.

17. Blondeau P, Wapler C, Piwnica A, Dibpst C. Deux cas de syndrome de la veine cava superierure trates chirurgicalement avec succes, l'un par desobstruction, l'autra par greffe. *Arch Mal Couer* 1959; 52:504.

18. O'Neill TH. In discussion of Scannel, J.C. and Shaw, R.S.: Surgical reconstruction of the superior vena cava. *J Thor Surg* 1954; 28:163.

19. Templeton JY. Endvenectomy for the relief of obstruction of the superior vena cava. *Am J Surg* 1962; 104:70–76.

20. Breslau RC, DeWeese JA. Successful endophlebectomy of autogenous venous bypass graft. *Ann Surg* 1965; 162:251–254.

21. Gloviczki P, Cho JS. Surgical treatment of chronic deep venous obstruction. In Rutherford RB (ed.), *Vascular surgery* (5th ed.). New York: Elsevier, 2001: 2099–2165.

22. Puggioni A, Kistner RL, Eklof B, Lurie F. Surgical disobliteration of postthrombotic deep veins—endophlebectomy—is feasible. *J Vasc Surg* 2004; 39:1048–1052.

23. Garg N, Gloviczki P, Karimi KM, et al. Factors affecting outcome of open and hybrid reconstructions for nonmalignant obstruction of iliofemoral veins and inferior vena cava. *J Vasc Surg* 2011; 53:383–393.

24. Meissner MH, Eklof B, Smith PC, et al. Secondary chronic venous disorders. *J Vasc Surg* 2007; 46(Suppl S):68S–83S.

25. Neglen P, Raju S. In-stent recurrent stenosis in stents placed in the lower extremity venous outflow tract. *J Vasc Surg* 2004; 39:181–187.

26. Raju S, Darcey R, Neglen P. Unexpected major role for venous stenting in deep reflux disease. *J Vasc Surg* 2010; 51:401–408.

27. Raju S, McAllister S, Neglen P. Recanalization of totally occluded iliac and adjacent venous segments. *J Vasc Surg* 2002; 36: 903–911.

28. Lugli M, Guerzoni S, Garofalo M, Smedile G, Maleti O. Neovalve construction in deep venous incompetence. *J Vasc Surg* 2009; 49:156–162.

29. Maleti O, Lugli M. Neovalve construction in postthrombotic syndrome. *J Vasc Surg* 2006; 43:794–799.

Index

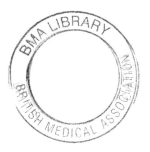